HEALTH OF THE NATION

HEALTH OF THE NATION

SOLUTIONS

THAT MAKE EVERYONE

A WINNER

VINCENT ANKU, M.D.

ISBN 0-9647741-0-0

Published by Achilles Publishers, Inc.
Cleveland, OH

Copyright 1994, 1995 by Vincent Anku, M.D.
Reproduction or publication of the content in any manner, without
express permission of the publisher, is prohibited. No liability is assumed with respect to the use of the information herein.

First printing, 1994.
Second revised edition, February 1995.
Printed in the United States of America.

Typography and design by Lasergraphics, Seattle, WA.

I DEDICATE THIS BOOK TO MY LATE MOTHER

AND TO ALL MOTHERS WHO ARE COMMITTED TO THE

PHYSICAL, MENTAL, ECONOMIC AND SPIRITUAL HEALTH

OF THEIR CHILDREN.

FOREWORD

As a nation, and as an international community, we are witnessing the dawn of an era of health system reform—an historical epoch that will not be completed simply by the passage of reimbursement reform in the United States. This debate has enormous ramifications for individual health care, the practice of medicine, the competitiveness of businesses, and the viability of national economies. Health system reform, in one guise and another, will last for more than one or two years; it will progress well into the next century as physicians, patients, community leaders, clergy, policy-makers, and others craft governmental and private sector responses for better health care practices, increased access to care, greater affordability of care, and improved health behavior by our citizens.

Here in the United States, our health system reform efforts are limited by a paucity of consensus around key principles or goals, as our vision of reform remains fragmented and unfocused. Of course, as a nation, we need to implement health responses that will address the causes of our current crisis—a lethargic and burdensome regulatory bureaucracy, a malpractice system that discourages the efficient and effective practice of medicine, a health insurance industry that often excludes payment for treatment of pre-existing conditions and the shocking health disparities between the general population and our poor and minority communities. Other problems make our health system less than user-friendly, while virtually guaranteeing rapid health care cost inflation. We also need to find better ways and means to prevent illness and disability, and, when unavoidable problems strike, to utilize the most effective, affordable, and humane treatments available. We need to make the preservation and enhancement of health status a top priority for each person, for each health professional, for each educator, and for each policy-maker. Such a pro-active approach will help to maintain, and increase, the freedom, independence, and productivity of our citizens, while bringing all of us closer together as family and neighbors.

Effective health system reform requires a rigorous, fair, and thorough examination of alternatives, discovering the best solutions for the complex, interwoven problems confronting those we serve—our patients. I found such a dialogue in this book. Dr. Anku is to be congratulated for his singular contribution to our current discussion on the "health of the nation". His "prescriptions" seek to preserve the advantages of a viable health system—high-quality care, well-educated health professionals, patient participation in prevention efforts, economic incentives to control costs, and a high degree of physician/patient autonomy. It also helps to lay the foundation for the future—positioning long-term responses necessary to promote a culture that values good health and avoids high-risk behavior.

This is a very readable, important document. Readers will find it insightful and stimulating—a blue print that makes all of us "winners."

Louis W. Sullivan, M.D.
President, The Morehouse School of Medicine
Former Secretary of the U.S. Department
of Health and Human Services

ACKNOWLEDGEMENTS

I would like to express my gratitude to my colleagues, family and friends who have assisted me in this ambitious undertaking. In every successful endeavor, there are truly committed people who unselfishly give their best. I am particularly indebted to Patricia Baker who has been instrumental in the preparation of this text at every stage. Her tremendous contribution and dedication to this project has made it possible for me to complete this book. I am also most grateful to CaMille Rhoades, who has greatly contributed her professional writing and editing skills in countless ways.

I gratefully acknowledge the help of Drs. Daniel Menyah, Walter George and L.B. Grossman; Attorneys Kojo Agyeman and Chad Brenner; Russell Catanese, Cynthia Ferguson and Walter Denz for devoting their time to read the manuscript and offering useful suggestions. I deeply appreciate the help, guidance and considerable time Dr. C. Payne Lucas has given me during the preparation of the book. My most sincere gratitude goes to Louis W. Sullivan, M.D., a clinician of extraordinary ability and intelligence, for the excellent foreword.

I am greatly indebted to Barbara Peris-Draves, the able administrator of the Surgery Center, Cleveland, for affording me the invaluable opportunity to provide a very efficient and cost-effective oncology practice at the top-rated ambulatory surgery center of Columbia/HCA.

Special thanks to my publisher, my consultants—Dan and Sara Levant and Lasergraphics—and Karen Domke.

I am most grateful to Grinnell College and Cornell Medical School for the full scholarships awarded me to pursue a superior education and prepare me for an exciting career in medicine. It has been a pleasure to practice at Southwest General Hospital in Cleveland, which was rated in the top 100 hospitals in the country during 1994 by HCIA.

My sincere thanks to two colleagues, Martin B. Taliak, M.D. and Barbara Gubanich, R.N. who have made consistent contributions to my professional success.

My three children, Kwame, Khama and Kofi continue to be a source of great pride and encouragement.

CONTENTS

Chapter 3
THE ROLE PHYSICIANS AND HOSPITALS MUST
PLAY IN REDUCING HEALTH CARE COSTS 39

Chapter 4
A CALL FOR MALPRACTICE REFORM:
THE ROLE LAWYERS PLAY 55

Chapter 5
A LOOK AT OTHER HEALTH PLANS:
WHAT'S RIGHT FOR AMERICA? 77

EXECUTIVE GUIDE TO HEALTH OF THE NATION

by

Vincent Anku, M.D.

President Clinton has stated that he wants a health care plan that reduces costs and provides access for all Americans. There has been a great deal of debate and argument about how to achieve this goal. The reason it has been so difficult to achieve these twin goals is because most people are misdiagnosing the problem. You cannot have a cure for an illness if you do not have the correct diagnosis.

In this document, we have produced a concise and clear diagnosis and solution for the health care crisis of this country. The beauty about our solution is that it accomplishes these goals in a free market without mandates or any increase in taxes. In fact, it will substantially reduce the cost of health care immediately and also cure the health care crisis for the current and future generations. We have been able to achieve these objectives because we have dealt effectively with the disease and not merely worked around the symptoms.

The health care crisis in America is primarily due to excessive and unaffordable costs. Hence, any solution that deals with pouring more money into the health care system is the wrong remedy and would ultimately aggravate the problems. While there are many factors that are driving up costs, there are three principal factors that need to be dealt with urgently that would produce exceptionally beneficial results. These factors are: providers—especially physicians, consumers and the legal system.

The current system of review for physicians, who are responsible for ordering most of the procedures, does not work. We have suggested a novel approach that would be very effective, but at the same time, would not be unduly burdensome on physicians. It can effectively stop unnecessary procedures before they are performed. We also recommend that physicians be encouraged to help stop unnecessary procedures. At the present time, doctors who speak up when they observe a problem with patient care become victimized even though they are only trying to protect patients and have no ulterior motive.

Secondly, no cost containment will be effective if the consumer is not given sufficient incentive to bring costs down. Where these approaches of consumer involvement and incentive have been used, the cost reduction has been near miraculous. The savings has been about 20 to 25 percent over a short period of time in every situation. We have covered examples of these approaches extensively in the end of Chapter 5 and in Chapter 7.

Finally, there would really not be a very effective reduction in costs without vigorous tort reform. The legal system adversely affects doctors' behavior at every step in their practice. Chapter 4 deals with effective methods of rewarding injured patients.

Those who are primarily interested in the solutions should concentrate on the following sections: controlling doctors' behavior and hospital cost containment discussed in Chapter 3; tort reform measures in Chapter 4; and the Medisave plan presented in Chapter 5. Chapter 6 discusses the right and wrong approaches to cost control. Chapter 7 should be read in its entirety because it deals with the solutions and puts everything in perspective.

The question being asked about health care reform is how to pay for it. The infusion of new money is not necessary. There is already more than enough money in the system. Something is radically wrong when we spend one trillion dollars on health care, yet more than 37 million people are uninsured. The primary reason so many are uninsured is that the cost of health care has become astronomical.

Industry is already spending 50 percent of after-tax dollars on health care. This is a serious stumbling block to an improved employment climate. To impose employer mandates on companies who can ill afford the expensive premiums is an invitation to massive layoffs. I am not philosophically opposed to small taxes or mandates, however, I do realize that to leave virtually intact the conditions that are driving health care costs through the ceiling and demand more money be pumped into the system is not the solution to the crisis. Who ultimately pays for employer mandates? *The employees!*

In summary, I believe we have come up with a very brief manuscript that offers workable solutions to the health care crisis. Our plan is one of the few solutions that makes everybody a winner. It can guarantee immediate access and can immediately reduce the current cost by well over $100 billion if we implement the major prescriptions outlined in this book. This will lead to the most viable health care security for all Americans.

INTRODUCTION

A Consensus for Health Reform

Every day, every hour, every minute somewhere in the United States a life is on the line: the 32-year old pregnant woman diagnosed with breast cancer; the father of four who's suffered a massive stroke; the reckless teenage driver critically injured in an auto accident; the baby girl separated from her Siamese twin with whom she's shared a heart for seven months.

An amazing quarterback whose superior athletic ability allowed him to zigzag between the defense for 70 yards and jump six feet above the last defender to score a touchdown, had his knee torn to shreds through a violent attack by the defense. A year later, the knee has been completely reconstructed and after intensive rehabilitation he is able to thrill the fans once again.

A Minnesota farmer has his hand completely severed in a tractor accident. A medical team reattaches the hand—muscles, bones, nerves, tendons and all—and after extensive physical therapy, the farmer's hand is remarkably functional again.

In each case, and countless others where the odds of recovery are slim, world-class medical care made the difference. The good news: the United States has the best health care system in the world. The U.S. has the best medical facilities and many bright and talented physicians trained in the world's top medical institutions. America leads the world in the treatment of cancer and heart disease. We have the best trauma centers and research labs. Skilled surgeons accomplish remarkable surgical repairs. Biotechnical drugs perform unprecedented medical feats.

The bad news: the price of being in the medical forefront has become increasingly unaffordable. It is destroying and will continue to devastate the U.S. economy if unchecked. Most of us find it difficult to relate to expenditures of billions of dollars and percentages of GDP. The following graph vividly illustrates the real crisis at hand.

The Crisis in Health Care Costs

Costs are in bilions of Dollars

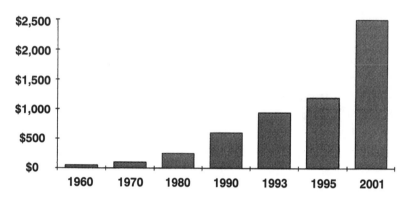

Data: Congressional Budget Office (*Newsweek* 10-4-93)

However, with all that has been written and spoken in the past year regarding the "crisis" in American health care and the need to reinvent the system, it is easy to lose sight of what is *right* with American medicine. An overwhelming majority of the American people are satisfied with their medical care and their doctors. Does any other profession or human endeavor provide this level of satisfaction? The question is—can we afford a system whose rising costs threaten to consume more and more of our economy, ultimately hurting every American? Nobody is questioning the quality of American health care. What is being rightfully challenged is its high cost.

The Crisis of Cost

Health care spending in the U.S. is the highest in the world. Since 1970, health care expenditures have grown at an annual rate of 11.6 percent—2.9 percentage points faster than our gross domestic product (GDP). In 1993, the nation's medical bill was nearly $940 billion, i.e. 14 percent of GDP. If we continue on this same course, by the end of the decade it could consume a staggering 18 percent of the GDP. Economists warn that in order to cover the health care bill we will soon have to cut into educational spending. Under the current system, we have to continue to raise taxes to pay for Medicare and Medicaid. Increased medical costs result in poorer contracts and compensation packages for workers. American companies forced to pay more for workers' medical coverage cannot compete in the global economy. This, in turn, causes more job losses in an effort by businesses to reduce costs. We are paying 35 to 40 percent more for health care than other industrial nations but, as a whole, we are not necessarily healthier.

One of the reasons health care costs are so staggering in the U.S. is the poor distribution of resources. A large segment of our population receives too much health care, much of which is unnecessary. Others get too little health care—or too much, too late.

Crisis of Future Cost

Amazed by the current expenditures? Future projections are even more astonishing. The aging population, technological explosion, violence and the AIDS epidemic only increase our already overwhelming costs. At our current rate of growth, 1993's health care bill of $940 billion will balloon to $1.2 trillion by 1995 and $2.5 trillion by 2001. Note, that by comparison, the entire federal budget for 1994 is $1.5 trillion. By the year 2011, the expenditure for Medicare alone will be larger than the Social Security and Defense Budgets combined. If the Medicare system is not bankrupt, it will be operating with an annual deficit of approximately $200 billion. Even more frightening is that by 2010 the first wave of "baby boomers" will be eligible for Medicare.

There are two major roadblocks to economic growth in America today. One is our national debt, a result of the reckless spending of the 80's. The second is rising health care costs and steadily increasing payroll taxes.

President Clinton argues that without system-wide health reform, all efforts to strengthen the economy and reduce the deficit will fail. The combined debt from the 80's, plus the rising cost of medical care, continue to compound the federal deficit. The deficit is the single most important reason for a future decline in the American standard of living.

Large corporations must keep health care premiums down to increase profitability and global competitiveness. Small businesses can't afford the rising costs of insuring workers. If forced to insure all workers at the astronomical cost of health care premiums today, many small businesses will close. The high cost of insurance is leading some companies to cut health benefits or provide very poor coverage, not only to future and current retirees, but to current employees and their dependents, as well.

In spite of these stark forecasts, there are still many who are leery of health care reform plans. They do not take the threat seriously or naively assert that there is no health care crisis. They fail to recognize that their own income and that of their children, will continue to stagnate or decline. And what's worse, they fail to see that they will face more bureaucracy and costs if our health care system is not carefully steered in the proper direction.

Anxiety abounds in the current health care debate. Hospitals and doctors worry that health care reform will prevent them from giving the best care to patients. They worry that the use of "high tech" medicine will be limited, that reform will stifle their ability to compete for business. Doctors also worry about added hassles, government interference and a sharp decline in some services.

Small insurance companies are scared at the prospect of having to fight it out with larger insurers like Blue Cross, Cigna and Aetna. Small business owners who, under some of the proposed health plans, would be forced to insure all of their workers, are worried about surviving in the marketplace. And patients—especially those who are employed and now have excellent health coverage—are afraid they may have to sacrifice the quality of care and the prompt service to which they are accustomed.

Certainly not everyone sees a successful solution in the proposed health care changes. But no one can deny that the U.S. health care system needs to be mended. Costs spiral upward, yet some 37 million Americans have no steady health insurance, while thousands more have meager insurance or fear loss of coverage. More than half of uninsured Americans are productive, employed workers of our society. Furthermore, according to Dr. Louis Sullivan, the former Secretary of Health and Human Services under former President Bush, a significant number of those without health insurance are workers and/or dependents of workers for small businesses. Yet many of these people do without health care basics like prenatal care, immunizations and cancer screening. Clearly something has to be done. While we may not agree with every element of the President's health reform package, the Clinton administration deserves credit for seizing the opportunity to open the long overdue dialogue on health care and for taking bold steps toward correcting the problem. All of the previous administrations even before Eisenhower have recognized the importance of dealing with our health care system, but none have been able to bring the problem to center stage—probably because it had not reached the crisis point.

The President and the First Lady have shown a great deal of courage and leadership in taking on an issue that most people think is impossible to deal with because of its magnitude. In truth, it is absolutely central to solving many of this country's other problems. We often hear people say "If it ain't broke, don't fix it." Well, our health care system *is* at a breaking point and we have to do something about it quickly. However, we must be very careful how we attempt to solve this problem or we may create a bigger monster.

The Federal and most state governments are moving at dazzling speeds to produce health care reform. Unfortunately, most of the currently proposed solutions do not adequately address the fundamental problems and will, in many ways, make the problem worse.

Over the last year, we have researched, studied and analyzed the medical care crisis and the many proposals for health care reform. We've conferred with many colleagues, listened to the politicians and their advisors, read the latest books on the subject and scoured over countless newspaper and magazine articles. Although some proposals offer excellent partial solutions to the health dilemma, we have concluded that the proposals offered so far —including the President's— will fall short of significantly reversing the health care crisis. Simply put, they fail to aggressively attack what we perceive to be the root causes of the problem.

The escalating costs of medical care can be attributed to three principle factors: physician behavior, litigation and patient demands. First, the behavior and practice methods of physicians dating back to their medical training leads to many unnecessary procedures. This includes excessive tests and inappropriate treatment provided to patients who are near death. Second, the constant threat of litigation results in doctors practicing defensive medicine at great cost to society. The third factor is what Dr. C. Everett Koop calls patients' excessive demand. Patients expect every possible treatment and the latest in high-tech medicine because they falsely think someone else is paying the bill. Hence, the consumer has no economic incentive to control spiraling medical costs. No amount of reform will reduce health care costs unless the consumer, i.e., the patient, is given a central role in bringing the costs down. This can be achieved by providing sufficient incentive and education.

The purpose of this book is twofold. First, we intend to clearly identify the problem—offering facts and figures to illuminate the magnitude of the health care crisis and demonstrate how this dilemma impacts individual and societal well-being. Second, we wish to provide government leaders, fellow medical professionals, insurance executives, entrepreneurs and working class citizens of this country a rational and painless, yes, painless, solution to the problem. A careful study of this manuscript will help industry and individuals alike, substantially reduce their own health care costs. We offer a solution that is based on an intimate, working knowledge of the American health care system. As previously stated, there is much that is good and "right" with America's health care system. Contrary to what the Clinton advisors believe, the system does not require a complete overhaul. Yes, it can stand for massive surgical reconstruction in some major areas and delicate fine-tuning in some others, but certainly not a total restructuring of the entire health care system.

Consider, for example, a football team that has lost a few key players due to injury. The team is no longer on the winning track and something must be done to correct the situation in order to keep the season from becoming a complete failure. Is it wise for the owner and the head coach to get rid of all or most of the players and start over with a brand new team? Or would it be more prudent to develop the strengths of the existing players, securing a tough running back and a good wide receiver to work with each other in the most effective manner?

In the chapters that follow, we will reveal just how we can genuinely reduce health care costs without wreaking havoc on our system—most importantly, without mandates or raising taxes—and yet provide coverage for *all* Americans. These solutions will help individuals, insurance companies, employers, hospitals and above all, the government, to reduce their share of escalating health care costs.

CHAPTER 1

The Growth of Health Care Costs and Its Impact

In this opening chapter, we provide what may appear to be an overwhelming amount of statistical information. However, these facts and figures are necessary to help illustrate the enormity and seriousness of America's health care problem. The data proves that there is indeed a health care crisis, and if not effectively dealt with, it promises to impact us all.

For the past 20 years, previous administrations and Congress have tried, with little success, to control the rapid growth of health care costs. Neither the regulatory policies of the 1970s nor the competitive policies of the 1980s have significantly slowed health care spending. Education has stayed at a mere six percent of Gross National Product (GNP), while the medical marketplace has grown from six percent of the GNP in 1965 to 13 percent in 1991.

We have allowed our system to plunge ahead without any judicious restraint and the effects are far more deleterious to the U.S. economy, American families and individual security than most people realize. Few people understand that there is an inverse relationship between the growth of medical spending and the growth of the economy and job security. Most Americans are satisfied with the care they receive and fear that cuts in Federal health care spending might lower their standard of care. However, when families are directly affected by the high cost of the health care system, it is only then that they find fault with the costs and financing of the system.

It was evident as far back as 1969—four years after the arrival of Medicare and Medicaid—that our health system was heading for trouble. We were warned by President Nixon then that if we continued on the same course, the system would face bankruptcy and our economy would be in jeopardy. Due to his immense concern, Nixon tried to introduce sweeping legislation to alter our disastrous course but failed to gain public and political support for his ideas. If there was cause for concern in 1969 when the U.S. was spending less than $75 billion a year on health care, we must certainly take notice of the situation in 1994, when we will spend more than $940 billion—more than three times the current defense budget.

If the present rate of increase persists, health care costs promise to surpass $2 trillion by the year 2000. Eli Ginzberg, Ph.D., of Columbia University brings reality to these incomprehensible figures by dividing our total spending for health care among the entire U.S. population. This translates into a family of four spending $30,000 for medical care in the year 2000, in contrast to $12,500 today. In light of the continued "graying" of the population, costly technological advances, urban violence and the spread of AIDS, this is a highly probable figure.

Simply put, our system of health care financing is no longer acceptable. We cannot afford the escalating costs of medical care. If it goes unchecked for only a few more years, as former Surgeon General Koop forewarned, the crisis will drive us into chaos. This chaos will not only have an impact on people who do not have insurance, but also on those who are now covered and think they have adequate and guaranteed insurance.

Good health care is a basic need for all people and with all that is available in this country, Americans have come to expect the best. Robert J. Samuelson, in an excellent article for *Newsweek*, succinctly identifies the dilemma we face. "Unfortunately, this feeling that people ought to have health care on demand fosters the illusion that health care is free. But someone has to pay, the someone is us and, frankly, we don't like that, either. The result is that our ideal health-care system is a logical impossibility." (*Newsweek*, 10/4/93, "Health Care, How We Got Into This Mess.") In order to resolve the dilemma of how to pay for good health care for all Americans, it is essential to understand the costs we are presently incurring.

Medicare and Medicaid

Medicare and Medicaid, two health care programs initiated by the government, are significant contributors to the uncontrollable health care costs. Yet, the reimbursement to hospitals and providers for these two government-run programs barely covers the cost of the services provided. Government programs are not known to be frugal and costs of government programs are always higher than projected. Social Security, for example, is a sound humanistic concept. However, the program is heading toward financial disaster because the government is spending almost everything it collects. Nearly 70 percent of current workers believe they will get less than half of what they contribute. Nearly another 25 percent believe there will be nothing there for them when they need it. People now perceive that the state of the Social Security system is so deplorable that 50 percent feel participation should be voluntary and they should have the option of investing part of their Social Security taxes privately. When former President Reagan suggested making Social Security optional in his 1980 campaign, he had to back off immediately because there was no support for such a "far off idea" at that time.

These same workers rightfully have very little confidence in the Medicare program. Even though there continues to be hefty increases in Social Security and Medicare taxes, these two programs face staggering financial crises. Social Security taxes are 25 percent higher on larger amounts of income than 10 years ago. In 1990, Social Security and Medicare payroll taxes were withheld on the first $51,300 of income. In 1991, payroll taxes were withheld on $53,000 of income for Social Security and $125,000 of income for Medicare. Not only have the base income levels for these taxes continued to rise each year, but the rate of taxation has risen steadily each year, as well. In 1994, Social Security taxes will be withheld on the first $60,000 of income and, for the first time, *all* income will be subject to Medicare tax at a combined employer/employee rate of approximately three percent.

Even with these high taxes, at the current expenditure levels, Medicare's budget may still be in deficit by 1994 and will be bankrupt by the year 2003. What's most frightening about this projection is that 78 million "baby boomers" will become eligible for Medicare in 2011. Even with the

Medicare hospital and physician payment reforms of the 1980's, Medicare costs have continued to climb. In 1980, total spending for Medicare was $36 billion; by 1990 it had reached $109 billion—tripling when the GNP has only doubled.

The three major social programs mandated, funded or administered by the Federal Government, namely, Social Security, Medicare and Medicaid, are all in financial shambles, or close to it. The Federal Government's own annual Trustee's Report, issued in April 1993, warns that as early as 1998, Medicare Part A (which pays hospital bills) faces bankruptcy. Even worse, the Medicare Part A deficit will increase seven times by the year 2000 and reach $16.5 trillion by 2070. The report of the Trustees, three of whom are members of President Clinton's cabinet, also warns that the fiscal crisis is so acute that immediate action by Congress is necessary for both short and long term goals. Between 1995 and 2000, Medicare Part A will lose $250 billion. The budget bill for 1993 may delay Medicare bankruptcy for three to four years and the Clinton Health Care Plan will probably do the same. The long-term outlook for the budgeting crisis of the Medicare system with all the current solutions, however, looks very bleak. At best, they will only reduce the long-term deficit by one percentage point. According to Roland King, Chief Actuary of Health Care Financing Administration, "The Trustee Report indicated that unless benefits are cut for Part A Medicare, revenues needed for keeping Medicare Part A afloat will require taxes to be tripled. This is how badly underfunded that program is."

No privately held corporation could survive by those standards of red ink. Efficient operation, cost containment and financial foresight are essential to the success of any industry. Health care is no exception. Various government program solutions to reduce the Medicare deficit have not worked satisfactorily. These solutions have been aimed largely at reducing reimbursement to hospitals, doctors and suppliers.

Medicare/Medicaid Spending

The Congressional Budget Office Report has observed that although recent Congressional efforts to reduce Medicare expenditures may be partially responsible for considerably slowing down the growth in Medicare spending in recent years, it remains a major problem. One of the most frightening parts of the health care explosion is the amount of money spent on Medicare and Medicaid. From 1965 through 1992, the combined spending of Medicare and Medicaid rose from approximately three percent of Federal expenditures to 16 percent. By the year 2000, this could easily top 20 to 25 percent.

In spite of the tremendous level of spending by the Medicare and Medicaid systems, these two programs are still being heavily subsidized by private insurance because the government does not pay enough to compensate providers for the cost of services provided to Medicare and Medicaid patients. The care provided by most specialists to Medicaid patients is essentially free since reimbursement through the Medicaid system is, in most instances, less than the cost of preparing and submitting the insurance claim. The billing system is so complicated and burdensome, that it is not unusual to receive several denials, requests for additional information or other delay tactics, with each of these correspondences accompanied by numerous pages of explanation, before a small payment is received.

The real inflation adjusted Medicare spending per enrollee has grown over 60 percent since 1980. The options of further increasing taxes or significantly reducing benefits are not easy choices. Taxes for Medicare have already risen significantly, particularly with the 1993 budget. From 1994 on, an individual earning $50,000 is contributing $1500 to Medicare each year. Over the course of 30 years, these contributions would accumulate to $138,000 even at a mere 6.5 percent interest rate. With the new law calling for Medicare tax on unlimited amounts of income, a person earning $1,000,000 is contributing nearly $30,000 a year to Medicare. Over the same 30 year period, this would accumulate to over $2.7 million. This amounts to a substantial subsidy by individuals to a failing system providing no guarantee that they will ever reap much benefit from their contributions. While the taxpayer is being hit hard, hospitals and some providers are also being squeezed and over-regulated by Medicare and Medicaid.

Medicare/Medicaid Underpays Health Care Providers

Reimbursement to hospitals cannot be reduced significantly further without causing severe financial strain. The Federal government's own data shows that Medicare currently underpays hospitals $10 billion per year. Many hospitals are barely breaking even due to operating losses on Medicare and Medicaid patients. These losses are recouped by shifting costs to private insurers. However, with the advent of managed care plans, private insurers are now refusing to pay higher reimbursements on services in order to subsidize Medicare and Medicaid.

After paying overhead and salaries to nurses and billing personnel, physicians too, often find themselves treating Medicare and Medicaid patients at a loss or close to a loss. Medicare payments to physicians are 50 to 60 percent of what private insurers pay. In many instances, the Medicare payment does not cover the expenses of the doctor. A neurosurgeon complains that Medicare's payment to him for surgical treatment of a typical carpal tunnel syndrome covers only the physician's costs for malpractice premium. Medicare reimbursement to physicians for chemotherapy drugs is now capped at the Average Wholesale Price. To control this expenditure even further, it has been suggested to limit payment to the actual invoice price, which provides no allowance for such costs as procurement, inventory and specialized disposal of the waste.

Ironically, while many cuts in reimbursement to physicians and hospitals are already being phased in, and many more cuts are being planned, proposals for new expenditures of an astronomical nature are being contemplated, such as adding prescription drug coverage for Medicare patients. While this is politically a very appealing offer to the multitude of Medicare recipients, the Medicare system cannot support the added financial burden. There are more cost-effective ways to provide medicine for those who cannot afford needed medications and, at the same time, substantially reduce the cost to those who are financially able to purchase their own.

America's Aging Population

From 1970 to 1990, Medicare costs have increased at an annual rate of 14.3 percent—significantly faster than the rate of 11.6 percent for all health spending and 8.7 percent for GDP. This growth is a result of increases in the number of enrollees, aging of the population, coverage of the disabled and those with end-stage renal disease and, most importantly, providing far too many more services than are necessary. Consider this astonishing statistic: one percent of the U.S. population accounts for 28 percent of all medical costs, while five percent are responsible for more than half the total. A large share of these cases are found among the 13.2 million Americans over 75.

Soon, many companies simply will not be able to afford to pay insurance premiums and will ultimately have to cut back or eliminate health benefits of their former employees. A survey conducted in 1992 by Foster Higgins, a consulting group, found that two-thirds of all companies surveyed had either reduced or planned to reduce health benefits for retirees.

This is illustrated dramatically by Unisys Corporation, which plans to stop paying health insurance premiums for its 25,000 retired employees by 1996. The computer maker said that keeping the program would have forced it to wipe out one-third of its net worth to meet new accounting standards and to pay $100 million in annual costs.

The Impact on American Industry

U.S. employers who provided health coverage in 1991 spent an average of $3,605 per worker—a total of $196 billion. Corporate America has seen health costs per employee double from $1,700 to $3,200 between 1985 and 1990.

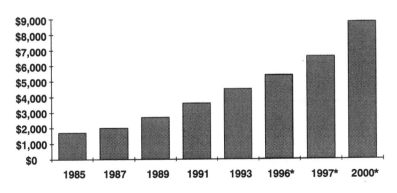

Average Health Care Premium per Employee

Projected Cost at 10% Avg. Rate of Increase

Data: Foster Higgins Survey, *Investor's Business Daily*, 5-20-93.

At the present rate, it will be $8,800 by the year 2000. The typical company's medical bill equaled *45 percent of after-tax profits*, an enormous handicap in the race against international competitors who bear no such burden.

Du Pont's per employee health care costs have risen 50 percent since 1989 and reached $6,000 per worker in 1992, as reported by Du Pont's Health Chief, Dr. Bruce Karrh, in an interview in *USA Today* (*USA Today*, 3/12/93). He noted that the rising costs are affecting global competitiveness for Du Pont's products. Du Pont's solution was a plan to double the employee and retiree share of health care premiums.

Avg. % of Business Net Earnings Consumed by Health Benefits

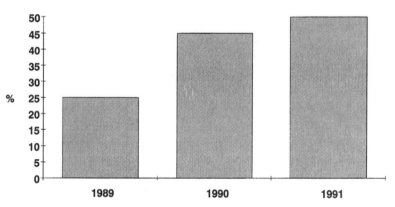

Data: Survey by Foster Higgins (*Investor's Business Daily*, 5-20-93).

Economic experts warn that the health care costs of our labor force raise the cost of United States-produced goods so much that we can no longer be competitive with Japan and other European nations. There is an increasing gap between Japanese and American competitiveness, especially in the auto industry. According to Chrysler's 1991 data, the first $1,100 of each medium-priced American car goes to pay the health care costs of the auto workers. General Motors spent $3.4 billion, or $929 for every car it made. The average Chrysler employee costs the company more than $6,000 in health benefits. It is a nightmare for American businesses, large and small.

As health premiums continue to soar, companies are left with no other choice but to stop hiring, lay off workers and/or scale back the wages of their remaining employees. According to a recent report by the Families USA Foundation, two million people lose their health insurance each month because they are either laid off or cannot afford the premiums.

Albert Shanker, former President of the American Federation of Teachers, shared some insights in an editorial in the *New York Times* in September, 1993. "…The health care costs always played a big part in our contract negotiations. The excellent program we had in the 1960's becomes poorer with each contract because of the increasing cost of health care. This leads to less money available to improve pay and working conditions. The health care cost is vital to teachers and education because the more we spend on health care the less money is available for education. With increasing unemployment, those who have excellent insurance may find that they have to pay more money out of pocket for meager coverage, if they are able to find a company that will insure them at all, if they suddenly become unemployed…"

Mr. Shanker compares the current health care situation to a story about a frog—which we all know can move and jump very quickly. If a frog jumped into a pot of boiling water, it would jump right out. It would get some blisters and burns but it would heal and recover. However, if the frog was put in a pot of cold water and the flame was lit under it, the frog would slowly adjust. He feels the water is getting warmer, but would not realize the water is boiling until it is too late. Mr. Shanker feels that perhaps we have not noticed that the "Health Care Water" is nearing the boiling point.

Problems Facing the Uninsured

In the past, most people weren't concerned about their medical bills because their insurance company picked up the tab. But with workers seeing higher out-of-pocket expenses in the form of co-payments and deductibles, a growing number of people are taking the risk of temporarily going without health insurance. As employers cut back on their employees' benefits, rather than see their paychecks shrink, workers are dropping their coverage and praying that a medical crisis does not occur while they are not covered.

Our hospitals have become experts at increasing charges to ensure that they recoup as much money as possible where insurance coverage exists. The wide-spread practice of passing the cost along to paying customers is known as "cost shifting." When the uninsured patient cannot pay their bills, hospitals tend to charge higher prices to those who can. This cost-shifting results in astronomical and often bizarre charges for pain killers and other medical supplies. Until everyone can afford health care, medical costs will continue to spiral upward with well-insured patients carrying a disproportionate share of the cost.

Drug and Technology Costs

Any discussion of the growth of health care costs would be incomplete without examining the rising costs of biotechnical drugs and sophisticated medical devices. Undeniably, genetically-engineered drugs offer physicians unprecedented opportunities to treat illnesses.

The prognosis was quite poor for a 70-year-old patient who was diagnosed with a rare, very aggressive type of ovarian tumor. The tumor was huge and had attached itself to the bowel in several places as well as to the bladder and abdominal wall making complete surgical removal almost impossible. Yet the surgeon was able to remove all visible tumor. While she was recuperating, within four weeks the cancer returned with a vengeance, causing signs of partial bowel obstruction. On her CAT Scan, a large mass reappeared. After consulting with three other oncologists at Cleveland Metropolitan Hospital and The Cleveland Clinic by phone, the patient was placed on powerful sets of chemotherapy called MAID.

Due to the availability of biotechnology drugs which can stimulate the bone marrow to produce more blood cells, the patient was able to withstand very intensive chemotherapy treatments to destroy the tumor. When her white blood count dropped to 400 she was able to receive the marrow-stimulating medication as an outpatient. A few years ago she would have died of the disease within months for lack of adequate doses of chemotherapy and/or due to complications of infection, even with a moderate dose of chemotherapy. Two years later, the patient remains free of tumor and leads an active life with her husband. Most important, the quality of her life during and after chemotherapy has been remarkably good.

Though a vital component of modern health care, biotechnology is pushing hospital drug costs through the ceiling. During the past 25 years, the retail price of prescription drugs has increased faster than the price of most other health care services. Some of the high-tech pharmaceuticals currently on the market include erythropoietin (EPO), granulocyte colony stimulating factors (G-CSF), growth hormone (GH), human insulin, and tissue plasminogen activator (TPA). These drugs are used to treat anemias, low white blood cell counts, growth hormone deficiency, diabetes, and heart attacks. Their utilization in 1993, as measured in sales, reached about $1 billion for EPO, $500 million for colony stimulating factors, $400 million for GH, $250 million for human insulin, and $400 million for TPA. And still more expensive drugs are on the horizon.

The use of pharmaceuticals accounts for six to eight percent of the nation's total expenditures on health care. As drug prices continue to increase at six times the overall inflation rate—an increase of 128 percent since 1980—the debate between Washington lawmakers and pharmaceutical manufacturers heats up. Congressional critics and health economists point to the double-digit profit margins of drug companies as evidence of price gouging. They ask whether it is fair for drug companies to make big profits off taxpayers who funded the research for the products they sell.

Pharmaceutical companies counter that initial government grants don't approach the $230 million-plus cost of developing, testing, manufacturing and marketing a new drug and that most of their profits are plowed back into research and development of new drugs. They argue that government price controls and attempts to cap profits will make it harder to find breakthrough drugs and will deny patients potentially life-saving treatments.

Private and public spending in medical research and development (R&D) have exploded. Currently, industry invests 7 to 13 percent of their annual revenues in R&D. In the public domain, the U.S. National Institutes of Health experienced a growth in budget from $26 million in

1945 to nearly $7 billion in 1990. New technologies such as endoscopy, angioplasty and new imaging methods, underlie some of this growth. Other examples of high cost technologies are kidney dialysis and transplantation, megavolt therapy, CT tomography and cardiac surgery. These sophisticated procedures often require specialized and highly salaried personnel to administer them. Labor costs for hospitals are currently about 70 percent of total hospital expenditures.

Combine these high-cost technologies with an overabundance of facilities offering the same services—and competing for enough business to make it profitable to operate—and the result is higher costs per procedure. The National Institute of Cancer estimated that 2,000 mammography units were needed for the U.S. population in 1990. At that time, there were already 11,000 units in operation.

In Summary

AIDS, violence, poverty and improper personal health habits (alcohol, drug and tobacco abuse) have had a significant impact on health care growth. The national cost of treating all persons with Human Immunodeficiency Virus (HIV) rose considerably over the past year and will continue to rise over the next several years. Studies indicate costs will increase 48 percent from 1992 to 1995—from $10.3 billion to $15.2 billion. It is estimated that the average yearly cost of treating a person with AIDS is $38,300. The number of individuals infected with the AIDS virus in North America is expected to rise from 1.2 million in 1992 to more than 8 million by 2000.

Having pointed out the obvious consequences of continuing growth of health care costs, it is clear that a solution must be found soon. But before discussing the best way to solve our health care problems, it is important to first understand the reasons why the American health care system is in crisis today. We cannot hope to reach a viable solution without first recognizing the many causes of America's health care problem.

CHAPTER 2

Why America's Health System is in Crisis

America's health care crisis stems largely from patients' and medical providers' disregard of costs. Until recently, health care was the only industry in which the individual consumer made purchases without regard to cost. This strange phenomenon has evolved from the expansion of a system in which a third party, either private or government, pays the bill. According to data from the National Center for Policy Analysis, patients paid out-of-pocket for approximately 50 percent of total health care spending in 1960. In 1990, out-of-pocket expense for patients had dropped to 20 percent. With little responsibility for the costs they incur, patients tend not to act as prudent consumers.

Physicians maintain control of the decisions that lead to at least 75 percent of all medical expenditures. By and large, most physicians are very sensitive to cost if it must come out of their patients' pocket. But without the need to consider the patient's budget, there is often no serious attempt by the physician to make carefully selected and economical choices in the tests and procedures ordered for diagnosis and treatment.

This chapter will address some of the many factors contributing significantly to the health care crisis. Those familiar with these factors and the detrimental effects on the cost of health care in the US, may wish to treat this section purely as a point of reference for specific examples of the problems we must confront in bringing about meaningful and workable health care reform. To that end, the chapter is broken down into numerous sub-sections to allow the reader to focus on those sections of particular interest.

The rapid rise in health care costs probably began with the introduction of the Medicare and Medicaid programs in 1965. With the passage of these programs, the method of reimbursement was based on what it costs the hospital to care for these patients, plus a margin of profit. Big mistake! In this kind of system—where the amount spent determines how much money the hospital makes—there is no incentive to save money. It used to be the doctor who admitted the most patients to the hospital and kept them in the hospital the longest was the darling of the hospital officials.

Another major blunder occurred within the insurance industry. The insurance plans of the 70's and early 80's were designed to cover inpatient services. Outpatient services, such as x-rays and diagnostic work were not covered. Hence, it became customary to admit a patient to the hospital for routine tests to reduce out-of-pocket expense to the patient. In fact, patients often insisted on being admitted so that the tests would be covered by their insurance. Today, the major insurance companies' policies are written so that most diagnostic tests and medical treatment are covered 80 to 100 percent on an outpatient basis. Now many insurance companies make it almost impossible to admit a patient to the hospital unless they are very critically ill.

At the same time, the proliferation of patient-friendly insurance plans have too many people going to doctors for symptoms as minor as a runny nose. Insurance coverage gives us the illusion that someone else is picking up the tab, therefore, many patients are not concerned about the cost of treatment. Some insured patients tend to overuse medical treatment—especially hospital emergency rooms, the most expensive form of treatment. Many doctors act on the premise that if the patient has good insurance coverage, cost should not be a factor in diagnostic workup and/or treatment.

For many employed individuals and their dependents, 80 to 100 percent of their health care premiums may be paid by employers with pretax dollars. The low co-payments offered through managed-care plans (HMO's and PPO's) give patients no incentive to economize in their use of medical services. There are patients who seldom question the cost or effectiveness of recommended visits and procedures because, under most managed care and traditional insurance plans, they aren't liable for 90 percent of the bill.

The method of reimbursing doctors is also faulty and contributes to excessive health care costs. Payment is based on usual, customary and prevailing fees, which means payment is based on what most of the doctors in the geographic area charge for a certain procedure. If there is a new procedure which is difficult to perform and requires a lot of training, the initial cost may be high. But as the technology becomes easier and the procedure takes less time to perform, the fee remains inappropriately high since there is no mechanism to cause a corresponding decrease in the charge.

Fortunately these examples of disincentive to reduce cost have been drastically changing in the past two to five years and will continue to change with or without government intervention due to extreme pressure by industry on private insurers and managed care plans. Still there are many other problems that continue to plague the U.S. health care system. It is impossible to address them all in the confines of this book, therefore we will focus only on those factors which appear to be major contributors to America's health care crisis.

Technology: The Number One Driver of Health Care Costs

Advances in technology over the past 30 years have dramatically changed the world. Medicine is no exception to this exploding development of technological tools and abilities. Many remarkable and highly useful procedures which are commonplace today were unheard of or extremely high-risk in the early 60's. Cardiac by-pass surgery even in the early 70's carried a significantly higher risk and was performed less often and with poorer results than it is today. Angioplasty can now safely open up clogged arteries for many patients. Much of the diagnostic testing capabilities available today, such as CAT scan, ultrasound and NMR, were non-existent 20 to 30 years ago. The introduction of Tagamet in the late 1970's has given many patients relief from stomach and duodenal ulcers without resorting to surgery to remove a great deal of their stomach and enduring all the ensuing complications.

This development has helped medical care in the U.S. to become the finest available in the world. VIP's from many other countries seek top-notch care in recognized American institutions such as The Mayo Clinic, The Cleveland Clinic, Scripps Cancer Institute, Sloane Kettering, Johns Hopkins Hospital, Massachusetts General and New York Hospital, to name a few. Americans have become accustomed to demanding and getting the best that technology has to offer—cost notwithstanding.

However, high level technologies have escalated the costs of health care tremendously. Ken Terry, Senior Editor of *Medical Economics*, called technology "the biggest health care cost driver of all" in the March 21, 1994 edition. He says that as medical advances continue to push costs up, more rationing will be required. Doctors will be the ones to inform their patients about these decisions. He also noted that politicians fail to tackle the role of technology in the health care debate because that would involve the "R" word—rationing—which does not win elections. Dr. Mark Pauly, Department Chairman of Wharton School of Economics in Philadelphia, states that in order to control health care costs, the growth of technology will also have to be controlled. He estimates that population growth and aging account for 10 to 15 percent of real growth and that technology contributes 50 to 75 percent of the remaining annual increase in health care costs.

In 1991, nearly 300,000 angioplasties to clear clogged arteries were performed. Unfortunately, arteries tend to clog up again, requiring repeated angioplasty and, in some cases, eventually lead to coronary bypass surgery. The number of coronary bypass surgeries performed annually has increased from 14,000 cases in 1970 to 400,000 in 1991. The number of CAT scanners, which provide an advanced form of x-ray testing allowing visualization of body organs, have jumped in the last 10 years from 300,000 units to more than 1.5 million units.

Nuclear Magnetic Resonance Imaging, also known as MRI, is a worthwhile, but expensive technology. The imaging machine, which enables doctors to view body organs at varying depths in great detail, comes with a price tag of approximately $2 million, not including the cost of building safety requirements necessary to operate the equipment. When there are too many expensive machines in operation in any geographic area, the operating costs per unit go up. The per procedure cost is increased to cover acquisition and basic operating expenses. The U.S. currently has about 3.5 MRI scanners per million people. By comparison, Germany has about one MRI scanner per million people and Canada has about 0.5 MRI scanners per million people. The extremely low level of availability in Canada may account for the influx of Canadians to the U.S. for more prompt testing.

Sophisticated and expensive laboratory equipment allows on-the-spot testing with minimal intervention by the operator. America is a society accustomed to instant gratification of demands. The easy availability of a vast array of laboratory tests have enabled patients' demand for instant answers to be met.

Physicians tend to overutilize the available technology for various reasons. First of all, advanced technology is employed because it is so easily available. Doctors are taught to respond to specific situations in specific ways. They are trained to leave no stone unturned in their search for the correct diagnosis. Secondly, the threat of malpractice fosters the pursuit of many possible, but unlikely, causes for the patient's symptoms. Finally, patients want and expect to have everything done for them and their families. An injury such as a knee sprain, can be accurately diagnosed over 95 percent of the time without the use of an MRI. In fact, the diagnosis can usually be made by physical examination alone. However, the use of various tests provides more concrete records and gives the physician the sense, whether valid or not, that he has protected himself from lawsuit in the unlikely event of misdiagnosis.

Aging Population

One of the major factors of increasing health care costs is the aging population. Estimates indicate that population growth and aging account for 10 to 15 percent of growth in health care costs. Our elderly are living longer because of the high level of technology and the advanced care they receive. Since life expectancy is increasing, the need for medical care continues to increase. The older the population, the more medical ailments they develop and the more medical attention they require. The health costs, of course, increase proportionately.

Once patients reach 65, the need for medical care increases rapidly.

Fortunately, many people over 65 are in excellent health. By age 70 to 80, medical needs have become even greater. The number of people over age 65 is growing and the proportion of patients aged 80 and older is increasing more rapidly than any other group. The implications for the health care industry are obvious. Since this segment of the population is growing and requiring more services, these services must be subsidized by the shrinking population of younger, working people.

Many of the nation's 13.2 million citizens over 75 receive unlimited access to high-priced doctors and technology, paying only a small fraction of the cost. For the elderly, hospital premiums are paid by the payroll taxes of others, and physician services are predominantly paid by general revenues. In 1993, the maximum Medicare premium was $32 a month, no matter what the recipient's income.

The cost incurred for the nearly 530,000 hip surgeries performed in 1990 was $9 billion. This was a four-fold increase in the number of these surgeries since 1980. Cataract operations have become the largest single-item consumer of Medicare dollars.

Nearly half of all Medicare dollars are consumed in the patient's last year of life, while 28 percent of Medicare expenditures fund the last four weeks of the patient's life. The sad truth is, we are spending the bulk of our medical resources on patients who are suffering from irreversible conditions. And what's worse, all this expense does not necessarily make their last few days any more comfortable or peaceful, according to Dr. D. A. Deutschman, former President of the Cleveland Academy of Medicine.

Despite attempts to reduce its expenditures, the Medicare system is still facing bankruptcy. Because the Medicare system consumes so much of our resources, it is the obvious target of attempts to cut spending. However, further reductions in payment levels to hospitals and doctors will not alleviate the basic underlying problem of fewer and fewer workers supporting ever increasing numbers of retirees.

In theory, our aged citizens have contributed substantially to the Medicare insurance pool all of their working lives and now expect to tap into those funds through health care benefits. In reality, by the time they reach retirement age their contribution has been consumed.

Glen H. Gronlund, speaking for the Ohio Presbyterian Retirement

Service, observed that as we age, we eventually reach a point where we need assistance, no matter how healthy and independent we may be. Research shows that about 12 percent of people who are age 65, require some assistance with things like transportation, housekeeping, preparation of meals, shopping, medication or home health care. Among the people over 75, the percentage needing assistance grows to 37 percent. And 70 percent of people over 85 need some sort of assistance. The government has promised our seniors that they will have insurance coverage for these sorts of services. Although these services are desirable, there is no money to pay for them at present.

Poverty

Poverty is a universal and constant predictor of poor health, even more than personal habits. Lack of educational awareness and lack of timely access are also important contributors to the spiraling cost of health care. Dr. Louis Sullivan, in his April, 1990 address to the American Surgical Association in Washington, correctly pointed out that concern about access to care for the working poor and uninsured is justifiable. Yet, the vast majority of citizens get medical care because of the medical code of ethics and government regulations. The care provided may not be as timely, but those who seek treatment largely get the care they need.

However, poor people often do not consider medical care a top priority and, therefore, do not seek treatment until they can no longer withstand the pain or suffering of their condition. Unfortunately, by this time, it is often too late. The lack of adequate routine and preventive care is a significant factor in driving up the costs of health care for the economically disadvantaged. It places a tremendous burden on an already stressed health care system. Dr. Paul Berk, M.D. of New York's Mt. Sinai School of Medicine, comments that the cost of emergency room visits and hospitalization for the poor far exceed the cost of preventive office care.

Without proper routine and preventive services, the poor in America seek medical help only when they are severely ill. They routinely show up in the emergency room for treatment—and in most cases, are admitted to the hospital. When they are gravely ill, no amount of expense is spared to take care of these individuals. A fraction of the cost could have been spent in basic health care if it had been provided before the patient became so acutely ill.

A pertinent example is an asthmatic patient. An average middle-class patient with asthma, who sees a lung specialist or family doctor on a regular basis, can avoid a serious asthmatic attack and continue day-to-day life with little interruption. If the asthma patient has a respiratory infection which might exacerbate the asthma, the patient visits a doctor's office. The physician renders appropriate antibiotic treatment, before the situation becomes urgent.

On the other hand, a poor patient is more likely to go without routine care, or prescribed medications. This patient will likely have many more acute complications and is more likely to be treated in the emergency room and/or hospitalized more frequently for acute asthmatic symptoms. These, in turn, may eventually lead to a long-term disabling lung impairment.

Failing to provide adequate routine care for the poor affects everybody. First of all, because the poor under-utilize available medical care, they become chronically and more severely ill, thus, diminishing the quality of their lives as well as their ability to maintain employment. They become an economic burden on their families and society and increase the strain on the health care system.

Contrary to what some believe the poor do not entirely lack access to health care. The problem is that they have the most access when they are critically ill. At this point, the state or the government says the hospitals must provide free care. We know that Medicaid does not come close to covering the full cost of the patient's care. If every hospital was reimbursed for all services at Medicaid rates, they could not function and would be forced to close their doors. In areas where the hospitals take care of large numbers of welfare patients, especially in the inner city, the cost is shifted to private insurance companies.

It is obvious that those persons who are working are being taxed directly or indirectly to cover the cost of those without adequate insurance coverage. This is a disguised tax in the form of higher insurance premiums to cover the cost of providing care for those who are not able to contribute to their own insurance coverage. Passing these costs along to the working population results in diminished pay raises or higher taxes. Dr. Berk questions the wisdom of structuring taxation to provide care in this manner and using tax dollars to provide expensive care to the poor when only a fraction of that amount could be used to provide care at an earlier stage.

Teenage Pregnancy

The explosion of teenage pregnancy is to some degree a uniquely American phenomenon resulting from the lack of adequate birth control knowledge and certain lifestyles. This problem is adding dramatically to the health care crisis and requires a solution urgently. Preventing teenage pregnancy and providing routine prenatal care would result in a tremendous cost savings. This particular group of mothers has little or no prenatal care which leads to babies with low birth weight and subsequent medical complications. Extremely low birth weight infants are often premature and are generally critically ill. Their care may require a tremendous amount of resources. When these babies are born in critical condition, all available technology is employed to care for them.

Due to the large numbers of infants born to teens and low-income mothers in the U.S. and the dismally poor survival rates of these infants, the U.S. ranks 21st in terms of infant mortality out of 24 nations ranked by the Organization of Economic Cooperation and Development. This is unacceptable for a country that has the best health care system, the best technology and the most highly-trained doctors in the world.

The fact is, many of these children have little chance of survival. For those that do survive, the cost of caring for each one of these extremely low birth weight infants can reach $2500 per day for the one to four month hospital stay these seriously ill babies require. The cost of taking care of them for life with their considerable handicaps and developmental problems, becomes another burden on the vanishing resources of society. This is a social problem. No health care reform policy or legislation will reduce the burden of teen pregnancy on our health care system if it does not adequately deal with the social problems that foster teen pregnancy.

It is incredible that society is so polarized and preoccupied with the survival and so-called murder of unborn children. This same segment of our society goes to great extremes to prevent abortions, yet does not make a genuine effort to ensure the survival of infants who are born healthy but die from preventable causes. It is a waste of our talents for society to be so divided and to spend so much energy and human resources fighting over the survival of unborn children. This fighting leaves little time to attend to the welfare and survival of children who are suffering and dying because of poverty, drugs, violence and lack of basic care.

The Surgeon General, Dr. Joycelyn Elders, is correct when she says she has never seen a person who needed an abortion if they are not pregnant. Once again, it is essential that we go to the source of the problem and try to correct it rather than spend our energies fighting each other at the point where we really cannot have much impact. It would make a lot more sense and save a lot of health care dollars if the pro- and anti-abortion camps could get together and find a way to direct their energies toward reducing teenage pregnancy by at least 50 percent by 2000. This, in turn, would substantially reduce the need for abortion and save a considerable amount of health care resources. There should be mutually acceptable ways that both pro- and anti-abortionists can reduce teen pregnancy by 50 percent by the year 2000.

It is absolutely essential for physicians to recognize the connection between socioeconomic conditions and health. The success of medical treatment for many people will be determined not only by the prescribed treatment but, in large part, by society's success in attacking and overcoming the effects of poverty and lack of education. Providing access to care is only a small portion of the solution. Many pregnant teens have some access to health care but fail to use it.

Poor childhood immunization rates are partly a result of lack of access, but lack of parents' education about the importance of childhood immunization is also a significant factor. When these children develop serious viral infections with complications such as encephalitis or meningitis, considerable resources are required to care for them. In spite of medical intervention at this point, the patient might develop permanent brain damage and require life-long care which, again, becomes a disproportionate consumer of the society's shrinking resources.

Education and Economic Status

Providing access to health care will do very little to improve the health of the underclass unless it is accompanied by access to better education and jobs. In many cases, access to medical care is available but people are not aware of it or choose not to take advantage of it. Even if they are aware of their options, they have other pressing needs that take priority in their daily lives. There is the very real probability that the health care of a substantial number of people will not be improved by simply funding a program to provide universal access to care.

The National Center for Health Statistics calculated a 23 percent increase in life expectancy between 1930 and 1965, while health care spending showed a negligible increase during that same period. From 1965 to the present time however, health care spending has dramatically increased with only a seven percent increase in life expectancy. John Merline (*Investor's Business Daily*, 5/13/93) calls attention to several independent studies all reaching the same conclusions regarding the strong connection between health, education and economic status. He questions the rationale for increased spending to improve access to health care when funds directed at stimulation of economic growth and more effective education might actually be more beneficial to the health status of our nation's poor.

Dr. Leonard Sagan, M.D., author of *The Wealth of Nations*, finds in his research that increases in life expectancy are often the result of increased wealth. Victor Fuchs, an economist from Stanford University, has concluded from his studies of health factors, that countries now providing universal access to health care, have not improved the differentials in health outcomes between upper and lower socioeconomic groups.

For example, he cites that infant mortality in the lowest socioeconomic group in Great Britain under National Health Insurance is still twice as high as the rate for the highest socioeconomic group—the same as before national health care was established. Even poor patients receiving the same medical care as their counterparts living in a more stable economic environment fare worse in terms of survival.

The *British Medical Journal* reported in the May 1, 1994 edition that poorer people in northern England are dying at about the same rate they did in the 1940's and early 1950's. The health of the wealthy greatly improved from 1980 to 1990, while the opposite is true for the poorest. Dr. Peter Phillimore of Newcastle University, co-author of the report, stated that this is the first time since 1930 that the death rate has increased, even in this group of poor patients. Their study found a strong link between health, socioeconomic status and employment. They concluded that public health is more strongly linked with material conditions and unemployment than individual behavior. They also showed that the average life expectancy of the poor in England has slipped from 12th in 1970 to 17th in 1990 among countries of the Organized Economic Cooperative Development.

Liz Hunt, Medical Correspondent for *The Independent* (4/28/94) commented that forty years of progress in public health had virtually no impact on the poorest people in northern England since they are dying at the same rate they did 40 to 50 years ago. Labor Party spokesman, David Blunkett, says his party recommends spending more health care resources in the underpriviledged areas of the North and inner cities as a solution to these widening health disparities. Here in the U.S., former Surgeon General C. Everett Koop has likewise noted that poverty is at the root of most public health problems.

It becomes glaringly apparent that the patient's living conditions can seriously undermine the benefits of good medical care. Higher levels of education, however, improve the patient's use of available care and promote healthier lifestyles. Providing better education and opportunities for economic growth, along with increased access to health care, is essential if we are to achieve any significant and lasting improvement in the health of our country's poor population and subsequently reduce the burden of their care on the system.

Destructive Lifestyles

We must acknowledge the fact that many Americans live destructive lifestyles which tremendously tax our health care system. Despite warnings, people continue to abuse their bodies with alcohol, drugs, tobacco and food. They ignore their health until a medical crisis occurs. Dr. C. Everett Koop commented in a commencement address to the Cornell Medical College Class of 1992 that, "Patients and our society can no longer afford to live as recklessly as they choose and then trust that rehabilitative and reparative medicine will patch them up."

Dr. Louis Sullivan remarked that physicians' role should be to first put their own house in order and then educate patients about preservation of health. While health care reform is important, staying healthy is crucial. Dr. Sullivan also observed that our success in biotechnology has, unfortunately, given our citizens the idea that they can do anything to their body and when they get into trouble, the health care system will fix them up. We must move away from that notion. Physicians should educate patients and communities about what to do to preserve and protect their health, he added.

In his November, 1990 address to Family Physicians, Dr. Louis Sullivan noted that cigarettes are the only legal product that, when used as intended, causes death. The hidden tax resulting from the costs society bears as a direct result of smoking amounts to $220 per person annually. He observed that although we have made some progress in reducing cigarette consumption since many Americans no longer regard cigarette smoking as glamorous, we still have problems with young people, minorities and women. Lung cancer has now replaced breast cancer as the leading cause of cancer death in women. Dr. Sullivan cited a 1990 article in the *New England Journal of Medicine* which states that women who smoke face three times the likelihood of a heart attack than those who don't smoke. Pregnant women have about a 33 percent higher rate of miscarriage, low birth weight and babies who die during infancy.

In developed countries, more than one-quarter of the deaths among people ages 35 to 64, are due to smoking-related illness. This information was summarized in a two-part article published in *The New England Journal of Medicine*, March and April, 1994, written by Thomas D. MacKenzie, M.D. and Carl Bartecchi, M.D., from the University of Colorado School of Medicine. Cigarette and cigar smoking is extremely dangerous. The 1993 report from the Office of Technology Assessment in Washington, D.C. found that one of every five deaths in 1990 was due to smoking-related illness such as cancer, emphysema and heart disease. In 1990 there were more than 400,000 deaths caused by smoking-related diseases. These ominous facts have lead former Surgeon General Koop to call smoking the most important health issue of our time and the leading preventable cause of illness and premature death in this country.

Smoking was first linked to heart disease in 1940. It has been shown to increase the risk of stroke, heart attack and peripheral vascular disease. Smoking is also responsible for about 85 percent of all lung cancer and is linked to cancers of the mouth, esophagus, stomach, pancreas, bladder and kidney, as well. The death rate from cancer is twice as high for smokers as nonsmokers, and heavy smokers have a four times higher cancer death rate. Cigarette smoke also contains a compound called benzene which may be responsible for about 14 percent of leukemias. Smoking also leads to other serious chronic lung diseases. Smoking-related pneumonia, influenza, bronchitis and emphysema caused about 85,000 deaths in 1990.

There are also dangers to non-smokers who are exposed to second-hand smoke. Environmental tobacco smoke is now classified as a human lung carcinogen. There is increasing evidence that non-smokers living with smokers have three times greater risk of dying from heart attack and heart disease.

The effects of passive smoke are very harmful to infants and young children. According to the 1993 report from the Office of Technology Assessment in Washington, D.C., 17 percent of lung cancer in nonsmokers is due to exposure to smoke as children. The incidence of respiratory infection in children exposed to smoking is also higher. Probably 150,000 to 300,000 cases per year are associated with exposure to smoke.

The cost of smoking is astronomical. Lost productivity and treating the smoker's diseases cost $65 billion in 1985. Another $110 billion is spent as a direct result of alcohol and drug abuse. Smokers are absent from work nearly seven more days per year than non-smokers. If Americans lived healthier lives, more funds would be available to take care of other crucial needs.

Various proposals have been suggested to curb smoking. The most significant of these is to help teenagers stop smoking and keep them from taking up the habit. About 80 to 90 percent of smokers start as teenagers, and every day an estimated 3,000 teens start smoking. Approximately six million smokers are teens and another 100,000 smokers are younger than 13 years old. It has been argued that the advertising and promotional events sponsored by the tobacco industry have intensified tremendously since the 1969 television advertisement ban. Much of this advertising has been aimed at children and teenagers. Consequently, surveys show that the number of six-year-old kids who know Joe Camel is almost identical to the number of kids who recognize Mickey Mouse. While the percentage of adults who smoke had been steadily declining since 1973, it leveled out at about 26 percent of the population according to 1991 figures available from the Report of the Advisory Committee on Smoking. Most current smokers are between the ages of 25 and 44.

Keith Henderson's interview with Joseph Califano, former Secretary of Health, Education and Welfare under President Carter, in the *Christian Science Monitor* (3/23/94), discusses the relationship of smoking to health care reform. Mr. Califano said that any effort to contain health care costs in the United States is doomed to failure unless it mounts an all out attack on substance abuse. He went on to state that a minimum of $140 billion of the nearly $1 trillion spent on health care last year can be attributed to drug abuse, both legal and illegal. He believes this may be a minimum estimate because it includes only the costs for illness and accidents experienced by people who are actually using drugs, including alcohol and tobacco. His figures do not include the huge costs for the secondary victims.

Most experts feel that if we can help kids get through the teenage years without smoking it would make a significant impact on the number of smokers. Hardly anybody starts smoking as an adult. Mr. Califano also felt that the recent studies have confirmed that tobacco use is closely tied to the use of other drugs. Furthermore, the use of tobacco also has a link to levels of education. It was shown in a recent CDC report that nearly one-third of people with less education smoke, compared to only 14 percent of the more educated segment of the population.

According to Drs. MacKenzie and Bartecchi, "Tobacco use has exacted a tragic toll on U.S. population. Every segment of our society suffers the consequence of these addictive products including a disproportionate effect on children, women and minorities. The human economic costs of tobacco use to our society are overwhelming. A uniform ban on tobacco advertising and an increase in the number of laws against smoking in public places, more aggressive public education and higher taxes on cigarettes would diminish some of the human tragedies and tobacco use."

Everywhere in the United States there are assaults on the use of tobacco. However, we must find a more effective way of helping people who desperately want to quit smoking but are having a hard time doing so. In addition, we need to help teenagers quit smoking or keep them from starting in the first place. Reducing the number of smokers will have an enormously beneficial effect on the health care system.

There are still other ways in which our behavior patterns adversely affect our health. While a large segment of Americans, especially the young, are very health conscious, many Americans don't exercise and are overweight. The diets of many Americans are too high in fat and sugar. We consume too many "convenience foods," high in calories and low in nutrition. "Fine dining" translates into large portions of excessively rich foods. Our diets contribute to a higher incidence of several types of cancer. Lack of proper exercise compounds the problems with our diet. Being overweight and the lack of physical fitness are important factors in heart disease, high blood pressure and many other illnesses.

Violence

Violence has become a major factor in escalating health care costs in the U.S. Although people don't typically think of violence when considering the problems facing our health care system, it is a serious health care issue that needs to be dealt with in an intelligent, rational, pragmatic and compassionate manner. Dr. Louis Sullivan identified violence as a public health priority which requires multiple approaches for solution and should not be the exclusive domain of the criminal justice system. It is not enough to try to improve health and well-being of children when they are under constant threat of violence and can't find a safe place to live and grow, he added.

Dr. David Satcher, Director of the Center for Disease Control, has pointed out the need to recognize violence as an important health issue. "If it's not a public health problem, why are all of these people dying from it?", noted Dr. Satcher in an interview by Peter Applebome for the *New York Times* (9/26/93). "I don't think you have to take anything away from the CDC' s historic role", he continued, "to say that if you look at the major cause of death today it is not smallpox or polio or even infectious diseases. Violence is the leading cause of lost life in this country today."

The Department of Health and Human Services' annual report on the nation's health found that the homicide rate for young black males jumped a staggering 74 percent from 1985 to 1989. The life expectancy for black males has slipped for six consecutive years due largely to increased homicide rates. Personal injury as a result of violence is estimated to cost society more than $100 billion annually.

Many Americans have become so desensitized to the violence around them that they are no longer shocked by it. Nearly every community has felt the effects of significant increases in juvenile crime and violence. In our inner cities violence has become a way of life. According to FBI statistics, between 1983 and 1992, the rate of violent crime increased by 57 percent, while the arrest rate for adult violent crimes rose nearly 50 percent. Young children observe the pattern of violence and copy it due to the profound lack of good role models close at hand. They view their situation with little hope for change. The value of a life is obscured by the hopelessness of their world.

Dr. Satcher believes that violence, substance abuse and teenage pregnancy are not the problems faced by our young people living among the self-destructive forces of inner-city life, but rather the consequences of the lack of hope for the future. He has substantiated his beliefs through the development of several programs directed at giving young people a sense of purpose. In a program started at Meharry Medical College where Dr. Satcher served as President, women addicted to drugs were helped to become drug-free. These same women were then allowed to use their first-hand experience to help other addicts change their behavior through "The Sisters Program."

Another program, "I Have a Future," directed at providing hope to teens, was so successful it is being copied in other cities. According to Satcher, instilling optimism and giving young people the sense that they can change their future helps them to deal with pressures of life around them. We could turn the tide significantly if we invest in education and provide jobs and purpose for these young people.

Author Bebe Moore-Campbell articulated this concept in a public radio commentary. She related a story of how young men traded their street gang status to join the South Central Panthers and dramatically changed their lives. She pointed out that these men were destined for trouble by their association with street gangs. Violence was the only way they knew how to define their manhood. The Panthers, however, now direct their energies toward fighting fires and other natural disasters. The role initially fills their need to define themselves in terms of facing danger and later provides satisfaction in discipline, a regular paycheck and pride in a job well done. The pattern is similar to bygone years, when young men living on the edge of self-destruction were salvaged and transformed by military life. Although the discipline of a military lifestyle won't turn all boys around, Ms. Moore-Campbell noted that "a lot of old guys could tell you '…If I hadn't gone to the army I would have wound up in jail.'" "Perhaps," as Ms. Moore-Campbell puts it, "we just have to find new armies."

California's jails are already filled to 180 percent of capacity. Forty other states have overcrowded prison systems. The recently popularized "Three Strikes, You're Out" anti-crime proposals nationwide threaten to add thousands of non-violent offenders to already overcrowded prisons for life at tremendous costs to taxpayers. It makes more sense to educate and employ our young people rather than spend $13 billion building more prisons and nearly $25,000 annually per inmate to keep them there.

AIDS Epidemic

The AIDS epidemic is wreaking havoc, not only in the U.S., but throughout the world. By the year 2000 conservative projections indicate 30 million people worldwide will carry the HIV virus. Some say the numbers could reach as high as 110 million. The implications of these projections are frightening and the devastating effects in terms of lives, families, economic productivity and financial costs cannot be underestimated.

The cost of HIV treatment is expected to rise 21 percent in 1994 due to increasing numbers of people infected with the virus and the fact that current treatments are keeping AIDS patients alive longer. Fred Hellinger, PhD., of the Agency for Health Care Policy and Research, (Blue Cross

Blue Shield, "Inquiry", 1991) estimates the cost of medical care alone for AIDS victims in 1994 to be $7.8 billion.

In addition to bearing the high cost of providing medical care for the AIDS patient, society suffers the economic loss of productive laborers in the prime of their lives, as well as the interruption of work performed by family or friends who devote time to care for the AIDS patient.

If we do not find a way to stop the spread of AIDS, the health care system will buckle under the strain. Dr. David Satcher encourages the view that providing people with the proper information to protect themselves is the key. And, as Satcher succinctly states, "...we can't let political, cultural or religious differences interfere with that."

Consumer Expectations

Aldona Robbins, Vice-President of a Virginia consulting firm, remarked that cost containment measures which do not directly affect the consumer do not have much impact. The demand side of medicine bears some responsibility for past failures to contain costs. This will continue to be a cause of failure under the proposed Clinton Health Care Plan. This is a very important concept because when patients are given true economic incentives to control their health care costs, the cost reduction is almost miraculous.

Patients today have grown accustomed to state-of-the-art care and typically expect miracles to happen through medical procedures. However, there is a large gap between expectations and the ability to pay for expensive and complicated diagnostic and treatment procedures. Studies reveal that as much as one-third of U.S. medical spending may be unnecessary. Hospitals, in their quest to attract and live up to consumers' high expectations, focus on the development of high-quality, high-cost technology rather than the development of good quality, low-cost technology. In addition to big ticket technologies, hospitals vie for patient dollars by expanding, remodeling and erecting lavish buildings, often in close proximity to other centers.

Any productivity gains over the past five years have been completely overwhelmed by the sheer number and degree of medical services provided. The cost of screening and follow-up care is often greater than any savings realized from early detection. For example, public awareness of prostate screening has been heightened by widespread publicity in recent years. Patients now frequently request this test to be done when visiting their doctor. However, while the screening test and early detection have merit, they are not without pitfalls.

A study of prostate surgeries in Wisconsin showed that the number of radical prostatectomies of men over age 50 tripled between 1989 and 1992. In 1992, the medical cost of this procedure in Wisconsin alone was $16 million. However, despite increased rates of detection, mortality rates have not improved. It is estimated that 29 percent of men in their 50's and 67 percent of men in their 80's have prostate cancer, although many are unaware they have the disease. However, only three percent have an aggressive disease and actually die from this form of cancer. Unfortunately, the positive predictive value of a prostate screening test (PSA) along with a digital examination is only about 50 percent. Therefore, many cases of prostate cancer will not be detected by the screen and rectal exam. In addition, benign prostate enlargement can often cause a false positive PSA test, so not all positive screening tests indicate the presence of prostate cancer.

In spite of these shortcomings, the number of PSA screens performed by Universal Standard Lab in Southfield, MI has increased over the past two years from about 100 to 200 per month to 6,000 to 8,000 tests per month at a cost of $40 to $50 dollars per test. We are not attacking these screening procedures but rather suggest doing research to find a more cost-effective way of using lab tests to provide doctors with more useful information, such as identifying which patients have an aggressive prostate cancer. It is also important to note that the use of screening tests without careful thought and appropriate clinical application by the physician can be costly and provide misleading information.

Administrative Costs

The high cost of administrative paperwork is taking a substantial toll on the American health care system. Between 1984 and 1988, the salary expenditures for personnel in hospital administration, data processing and medical care review departments grew 30 to 45 percent faster than salary expense for all workers nationally, according to data from the American Hospital Association's Monitrend. *Automated Medical Payments News*, a newsletter for the insurance industry, stated that $120 billion was spent in 1992 on administrative costs. As much as 25 percent of each medical care dollar goes to cover administration costs. These averages were unchanged in areas of the country with high enrollment in HMOs—indicating that HMOs do not necessarily impact any change in administrative costs.

The number of personnel necessary to accommodate all of this bureaucracy has also increased. According to a report by Dr. Steffie Woolhandler, M.D., et al, (*New England Journal of Medicine*, 10/5/93), using statistics published by the American Hospital Association, hospitals employed 435,100 managers and clerical workers for approximately 1.4 million in-patients on an average day, in 1968. By 1990, there were about 1.2 million clerical workers and managers for 853,000 patients. Addressing problems in the business of health care administration will save time, paper and mental frustration.

Excessive Paperwork. With nearly 1500 different health insurance companies, the number of different forms and requirements for the format and content of a bill for medical care are endless. All services and diagnoses must be translated into numerical codes in order to bill the insurance company. Not all insurance companies recognize the same set of codes and many have specific requirements as to the manner and sequence in which the codes are reported.

The Medicaid form required for a physician to justify the need for a bedside commode is four pages long. Medicaid issues a multitude of pages to detail the explanation of a minimal payment or make a payment denial and request further information. Medicaid frequently denies claims on the grounds that insufficient information was provided, when in fact the information was already provided on the original claim. These delays also drive up costs for providers by increasing the need for clerical personnel to respond to requests for information and follow up on delayed claims.

Many employee benefit programs waste time and money with inefficiencies that result from a basic lack of foresight and common sense. In order to pay their employees for time lost from the job due to illness,

General Motors requires a separate claim form to be completed by the doctor for each day the employee misses work unless those days are consecutive. Patients receiving chemotherapy treatments once a week must have a new claim completed by the doctor each week, even when the employer was notified in writing that treatments would be administered once a week for a specific length of time. Disability claim forms from the state are typically three to five pages long and ask for the patient's diagnosis and the names of prescribed medications in three separate places on the form.

Not only does form shuffling increase costs and generate paperwork, it also increases the time physicians and other medical personnel must devote to completing and filing forms and detracts from the time they are able to spend caring for patients. Often additional clerical workers are needed just to keep up. The 1988 *Journal of the American Medical Association* reports that an average U.S. doctor's office staff spends one hour per claim preparing, submitting and collecting payment from Medicare or Blue Cross. The survey also found that billing expense and overhead costs, excluding malpractice expenses, consumed 43 percent of physicians' gross practice income in 1988. Adding in malpractice expenses, which average 11 percent of income, pushes the doctor's overhead expense to more than 50 percent of gross practice income.

Switching from paper to electronic transmission methods will achieve savings in the cost per claim form submitted but the switch will cost more in other ways since not all insurers and providers are currently equipped with the necessary computer capabilities. Uniform requirements and streamlined forms, along with assistance from the insurance industry to facilitate more widespread electronic capabilities, can help to reduce paperwork costs and allow time to be redirected to productive ends.

Cost Containment Programs. Strict scrutiny of care and procedures by managed care programs requires a large number of people to administer. Utilization review has become the fastest growing segment of the health care economy. The gatekeeper concept has created an entire industry of administrative functions and personnel. Consider the duplication of utilization review and pre-certification departments at hospitals and most insurance companies. The system is arbitrary and inefficient with far too many people involved in the same certification process.

An orthopedics physician cited an example of a major insurer who required that patients seeking hip replacement be unable to tie their shoes before granting approval for hip replacement surgery. This criteria, as a standard for measuring medical necessity of the procedure has no medical or scientific basis. Review of a case is usually conducted by telephone. The reviewer goes down a list of pre-established questions. If the provider becomes proficient at knowing what sort of information the reviewer needs to hear, then the process has failed to accomplish its intent. If the provider does not answer the questions correctly, the care will be denied, although the true picture of the patient's case may not have been presented by the types of questions and answers exchanged.

A more valid approach to review, which has also been suggested by Dr. Robert Brook of the Rand Corporation, would be to form on-site review committees in hospitals to examine the need for procedures before they are performed. The current hospital-based review systems merely look at a few selected cases each month involving services that have already been performed.

Mandatory Second Opinions. In theory, mandatory second opinions are a sound idea. In reality, obtaining a second opinion has not been successful in preventing unnecessary procedures. Furthermore, second opinions on surgery have generated a substantial increase in medical costs, as well as a great deal of confusion for patients. In the first place, disagreement about a course of action does not inherently make one choice "unnecessary" or wrong. In addition, when a conflicting second opinion is given, patients usually do not have sufficient knowledge about the procedures and predicted outcomes to effectively discern which opinion is the correct choice for their situation. Scrutiny of the medical necessity and appropriateness of a procedure would be better left to a panel of unbiased reviewers.

Excessive Regulation. Government regulations also add considerably to the cost of medical care, often without achieving any real benefit. For example, the Clinical Laboratory Improvement Act of 1988 was designed by Congress presumably to protect the consumer from erroneous laboratory results. The law, which applies to some degree, to all types of laboratory testing was passed as a result of highly publicized problems with the reading of PAP smears. To this day, however, the regulations have not been fully implemented although all providers of laboratory services have been required to pay considerable funds to administer the regulations. Six years after the regulations were proposed, further modifications to make the rulings less cumbersome are still being contemplated by the Clinton Administration.

The required registration of a laboratory with the Federal government consists of completing a 12-page form followed by a five-page form asking the same questions in a different format. Remittance of a $100 to $600 registration fee and an inspection fee ranging from $800 to nearly $3000 depending on the number and variety of tests performed is required in advance. While payment of fees was required in 1992, many labs have yet to be inspected. Compliance with the regulations requires an array of charts, forms and documentation to prove ongoing monitoring of laboratory test results. While this is a worthy goal and quality control is a necessary component of any type of testing, generation of such extensive paperwork and regulation of even the most minute details, such as the format of the printed test report, is indeed over-regulation.

There has been rampant confusion about the regulations due to poor communication with providers and lack of consensus about interpretation and application of the law. Much of the confusion stems from the fact that lawmakers drafted the regulations with little first-hand input from technical personnel. Many of the proposed applications have been abandoned due to inherent contradictions and the simple fact that they just don't work.

The CLIA regulations are another example of a government program which is costing far more than expected and having great difficulty accomplishing its intended purpose. There is a clear need to protect the patient and ensure uniform, high quality laboratory testing. Therefore, we must carefully devise a better system to target the incompetent and dangerous elements in the laboratory business. Clearly the CLIA law is an over-reaction to an obvious problem caused by a few laboratory personnel. President Clinton is quite right in stating that much of this over regulation should be repealed by the current reform proposal.

So far we have discussed health care growth in America and its overall impact on individuals and society. We have pointed out some of the reasons for this staggering growth. Now it is time to focus on what must be done to avert the health care crisis.

CHAPTER 3

The Role Physicians and Hospitals Must Play in Reducing Health Care Costs

There is much that doctors can do to reduce medical costs in this country. Overtreatment and inappropriate treatment can consume vast amounts of health care dollars without providing any significant benefit to many patients. Overtreatment can cause further problems by exposing the patient to unnecessary risks and opening the door to other complications which, in turn, must be treated.

Both physicians and patients have earned a share of the responsibility for this costly and complex scenario. Many patients are not satisfied unless they receive all possible tests and treatments although these test may not necessarily help them. They expect—even demand—to receive some specific testing and medication when they visit their doctor. However, determining what treatment options are *appropriate* for the patient is the responsibility of the physician and it is his or her obligation to recommend the most appropriate course of action in a given situation.

On the other hand, there is a wide-spread impression that much of what physicians do is unnecessary. In a minority of cases this barrage of waste is fueled by greed, but in most cases, it is primarily due to physicians' inability or failure to implement other, more cost-effective procedures into their practice patterns, largely due to training and practice habits.

For example, until recently, the usual recommendation in many quarters was to perform a yearly colonoscopy on patients who have had colon cancer. However, this may not be necessary. A recent study in the *New England Journal of Medicine* (4/1/93) concluded that performing the procedure annually provides no greater benefit than if done once every three years, obviously with a few exceptions. With this type of vital information from well-controlled clinical studies, the doctor feels more comfortable performing the procedure less often.

Generally, more than 75 percent of all services are ordered by doctors. If doctors changed their practice patterns and performed only what is necessary for speedy diagnosis and treatment of the patient, health care costs would come down substantially.

Consider a situation which often occurs when a hospitalized patient is admitted with various problems and complaints. Several specialists may be called in to evaluate and manage different aspects of the patient's care. Each specialist concentrates on providing their specialty service to the patient, just as they have been requested to do by the admitting physician. And each specialist orders the sophisticated testing relating to his or her specialty. This proliferation of consultations is fueled by the malpractice system in the United States. Physicians limit the scope of their responsibility and thus liability, by referring the patient to a specialist.

For example, an elderly woman falls, fractures her hip and is admitted to the hospital for treatment. As part of the pre-operative screening, it is discovered that she has a slight anemia. Although this level of anemia is quite common in elderly patients, and could be evaluated by the family physician or surgeon, a hematologist is usually called in to evaluate and treat the anemia. Due to the woman's past history of congestive heart disease, a cardiologist is called in to evaluate the patient and give the OK for surgery, in spite of the fact that the woman is not in any acute distress. While recuperating from her surgery, the woman develops a pneumonia and a pulmonary lung specialist is called in to treat her.

With the exception of the surgery to repair the fractured hip, all of these problems could have been handled by the patient's family physician at much less cost. However, the family physician is often completely out of the picture by this time. There is usually a billing restriction on concurrent care by more than one physician, and the family doctor may not get paid for his services in such a situation. Consequently, no single physician is controlling the direction of the care as a whole. If any of the findings indicated a more serious or complex underlying problem, a specialist's expertise could be valuable in managing the patient's care. However, utilizing specialists to provide basic care is a costly but prevalent pattern that must be altered.

Doctors' Autonomy

There is possible danger in any professional having absolute autonomy—especially when it involves them doing whatever they feel is justified in the care of a patient. This can be costly to the system and may not always be in the best interest of the patient. Take, for example, the 90-year-old woman who has suffered a hip fracture. Prior to the patient's accident, she was bedridden and unable to walk. The question is, should this patient be subjected to anesthesia and surgery? The chances of her surviving such a serious operation are slim at best. And even if she does make it through surgery, there is a strong likelihood of her developing complications and dying in the hospital. In this case, and many others, a team of doctors would be able to independently offer judgment on whether the hip surgery is appropriate—given the circumstances. One should not view this as rationing, but as patient protection.

An article in *British Medical Journal*, May 1988, emphasized the need to limit unchallenged doctors' autonomy, especially in regard to cancer patients. Due to wide variation in treatment and judgment, it would be beneficial to patients and physicians alike to establish reasonable and practical practice guidelines.

Investigation of vague or non-specific symptoms is a difficult situation which often results in excessive and unnecessary procedures. For example, diagnostic evaluation of dizziness or fainting is often a costly path leading to no clear answer. Unexplained fainting or dizziness, known as syncope, is a frequent complaint of many patients visiting their doctor. Pursuit of a diagnosis costs an average of $23,000 per patient. In a study of 121 patients in a Pittsburgh hospital from 1976 to 1980, a clear cause for their disorder was identified in only 13 cases. According to the study published by Wishwa N. Kapoor, M.D., et al. (*Journal of the American Medical Association*, 5/21/82) EKG's, CAT scans, cardiac catheterization and cerebral angiograms are some of the procedures used to determine a cause for the patient's symptoms. The low success rate of finding the cause indicates that extensive evaluation of syncope is not cost-effective and specific accepted approaches should be developed describing what sort of testing is indicated and appropriate in ruling out possible serious causes.

Many high-cost procedures are performed without true need. Two studies released in the *Journal of the American Medical Association*, September, 1993 clearly show the futility of persistent cardiac resuscitation attempts. Out of 1710 cardiac arrest victims who were resuscitated by paramedics, only **nine** survived. All but one of those nine had significant brain damage as a result of prolonged oxygen deprivation. If the victim does not immediately respond to resuscitation attempts, an informed decision should be made as to when efforts to resuscitate should be stopped. According to the study by Dr. Arthur Kellerman, M.D. of Emory University in Atlanta, following this simple guideline would save $500 million to $1 billion annually.

Another study by Dr. Mark Thel of Duke University Medical Center, showed similar results. Of 146 patients who were resuscitated after cardiac arrest while in a surgery or general medicine ward of the hospital, less than 5 percent ever left the hospital. The average stay in the hospital after resuscitation was 459 days, most of which was spent in intensive care units on mechanical ventilation.

About 20 percent of permanent pacemakers are thought to be inappropriate, according to the work of A.M. Greenspan, et al. (*New England Journal of Medicine*, No. 318, 1988). One in every 500 people in the U.S. receives a pacemaker at a cost of about $2 billion annually. A 1988 study published in the *Journal of the American Medical Association* (JAMA) concluded that one-half of all coronary bypass grafting was performed for inappropriate reasons. The cost in 1988 was $3.5 billion. Another study published in 1988 in the *New England Journal of Medicine* indicated that two-thirds of all surgeries for blocked carotid arteries in the neck were unnecessary.

Is managed care the answer to controlling overutilization of high-cost procedures? A study conducted on seven major HMO (Health Maintenance Organization) systems in the U.S. indicates this is not the case. The study (*Journal of the American Medical Association*, May 1993) conducted by a group of physicians for the Health Maintenance Organization Quality of Care Consortium revealed that the number of unnecessary or questionable hysterectomies performed by doctors working for HMOs like Kaiser Permanente, who have no economic incentive in performing the procedure, is almost identical to the number of unnecessary or questionable hysterectomies performed by doctors in private practice, operating in a fee-for-service system.

Practice Patterns

Traditionally, it has been argued that physicians' financial incentives were the primary reason for the large number of unnecessary procedures. Interestingly, however, even in the HMO setting in which physicians' financial incentive has been eliminated, substantial overutilization is still evident. This belies the point that habitual practice patterns and training play a large role in determining what care will be provided. It becomes apparent that an HMO does not in and of itself control unnecessary procedures.

Most doctors agree that the things we do are mostly done out of habit, stemming all the way back to our medical school training. But by changing these wasteful and often ineffective practice habits, we can save at least 10 percent of what we are now spending on health care—money that could take care of all the poor and underserved, as well as reduce the exorbitant premiums currently charged to those with insurance coverage.

Immunodiagnostic testing to monitor patients with previously diagnosed cancers is a relatively new technological tool with rapidly expanding utilization patterns. In 1980, immunodiagnostic testing was just becoming available. According to a report by Frost & Sullivan, Inc., an international market research firm, sales in 1980 for these types of products totalled $14.3 million nationwide. By 1990, sales had reached $586 million. While many different types of tests were developed during that period of time accounting for the dramatic rise in sales, it is highly likely that overutilization is also occurring. It may be necessary to establish guidelines as to the recommended frequency of performing these tests. This will provide valuable information to the physician in the management and treatment of the tumor, while maintaining cost effectiveness.

Over-utilization of lab testing is frequently observed in many areas. The causes for this range from subtle to blatant. Often it is simply a matter of the physician's habits and training when faced with specific situations. Sometimes patients want certain tests to be done. Also the fear of lawsuit is an underlying motivator, consciously or subconsciously. There is the false sense of security that if more tests are done, there is less likelihood of a lawsuit for "missing" something that should have been discovered.

Controlling the Cost of Prescription Drugs

Contrary to what some in the medical profession believe, I contend that we can reduce health care costs without sacrificing the quality of patient care. One way for us to curtail costs is to take responsibility for deciding how best to use the available resources. No one can deny the enormous contribution technological progress has made in the effectiveness of medical care, but we must learn to use technology more prudently—and that includes prescription drugs. The way physicians prescribe drugs is as much responsible for spiraling pharmaceutical costs as is inflation in drug pricing. It's not uncommon for elderly patients to have a medicine cabinet full of prescription drugs—many of which are duplicates and worse yet, some that are never even taken. These patients often have a family doctor in addition to two to four specialists, all writing prescriptions in their specialty areas. The use of prescription drugs can be best managed and monitored by the patient's primary care doctor. The doctor can communicate with the other attending physicians and coordinate an effective drug therapy program. Furthermore, family practice doctors should be better compensated for their time-consuming work.

Doctors are largely responsible for the kinds of drugs purchased and the amounts used. Many hospitals have begun educating physicians on the merits of lower-cost drug substitutions and orienting them on how to assess the value of certain drugs. Hospital formularies, which are lists of medications that the hospital or insurance company prefers based on overall cost of the therapy for a specific diagnosis, have proven to be a useful tool in controlling costs. The physician is encouraged to provide only those drugs listed in the formularies unless there is a compelling reason to choose something else.

Misguided Spending

According to a 1989 survey by Dr. Robert Brook, M.D., Senior Scientist of The Rand Corporation, a significant proportion of the medical procedures analyzed in their study were unnecessary. If these figures are extrapolated across the board to all medical care provided in 1989, $400 billion could be eliminated from health care expenditures by stopping our misguided spending. Using 1992 Medicare data, David Foster, chief Statistician for HCFA, remarked in *Medical Economics* (3/21/94) that one out of every five inpatient hospital days was unnecessary. Hospitals could save $1.2 billion a year if that extra unwarranted day of confinement was eliminated. He predicted that within five years, most U.S. hospitals will be forced to produce low cost, high quality, efficient medicine that will drastically reduce such costs.

One of the most tragic examples of misguided spending surrounds the issues of terminal care. Nearly one-half of all Medicare dollars are consumed in the beneficiary's last year of life and 28 percent of all Medicare expenditures fund the last four weeks of life. These figures tell us that we are spending precious resources in ways that do not benefit the patient and may, in fact, cause them some suffering.

Knowing when to stop trying to cure a patient is difficult for family members as well as physicians. There are complex factors involved in this decision. First of all, it is often difficult, if not impossible, to determine when the patient is entering the final few weeks of life. The physician and the family are caught up in their efforts to try to "pull the patient through." Secondly, our inability as a society to face our own death or that of a loved one sometimes causes us to hang on too long. Fear of a lawsuit if the family believes treatment is stopped too soon—that not enough was done to save their family member—can also cause physicians to continue treatment.

In many situations, the family is completely at a disadvantage, and is unable to make the decision to stop treatment. They are unable to "deny" their loved one any possible hope for the last chance at survival. What the family often does not realize however, is that further attempts to keep the patient alive are only prolonging the inevitable. The consequence of postponing the patient's death is prolonged pain and suffering for their loved one. It is up to the physician to remove the burden of this decision from the family by recognizing when the time has come to stop treatment. The physician should make it clear that continued treatment is not in the best interest of the patient. Presented with this information in a caring, honest and straight-forward manner, few family members would demand continued treatment.

When talking to people about their experiences, nearly everyone—both lay people and medical professionals—has had some first-hand experience with what they considered to be unnecessary care. A doctor from Chattanooga told of an elderly family friend who had cardiac bypass surgery. Prior to surgery, the man's heart was so weak he could scarcely perform any normal activity. A MUGA scan, which measures the strength of the heart muscle, showed a result of only 25 percent. His heart muscles were simply too weak to function even if proper circulation were restored. However, the surgeon convinced the wife that the bypass was the only possible way to improve this man's quality of life. Not wanting to "deprive" her husband of this last opportunity, the wife agreed to the surgery. It should have been no surprise that the man did not survive.

An oncologist related the case of a prominent member of his community who was found to have a large lung tumor. Although there was much to alert the surgeon that the tumor was too massive and too close to vital organs for the patient to be a surgery candidate, the man was still scheduled for surgery. The patient's chest was opened, the tumor was deemed inoperable and the surgeon closed him up. The physician sent the man for radiation, designed to shrink the tumor, and scheduled a second operation. Although the radiation had failed to shrink the tumor sufficiently to warrant a second attempt to remove it, the patient was subjected to the second unsuccessful operation. Several months later, after two unsuccessful surgeries, the patient was sent to an oncologist after the tumor had spread to the brain.

A story, which I heard on the radio last year, described a woman, more than 80 years old, who was developing what appeared to be a gangrene condition of her foot. The doctor wanted to amputate the foot. The woman inquired as to what would be accomplished by amputation and was told that she could die without removing her foot. The patient calmly informed the doctor that she had enjoyed a long and pleasant life and did not want to live without a foot. The doctor was shocked that the woman would choose to die without trying to prevent the inescapable results. Were it not for this woman's strength and logic, she would not have been offered the option of doing nothing. Soon after, she died peacefully.

A gentleman from Washington State shared with me the story of his 80-year-old mother's experience with leukemia. Her doctor informed the family that her only choice was chemotherapy. The woman became so ill from the side effects of her first treatment that she had to return to the hospital due to extreme dehydration and infection. After a lengthy recovery, the doctor suggested another course of a half dose of chemotherapy. The gentleman asked the doctor what they were trying to accomplish in the treatment of his mother and if there was any possibility his mother's condition might improve. The doctor said he didn't know but that it was her only chance. The man told the doctor that if there was no decent chance of improving his mother's survival or quality of life, he would prefer to take her home and make her as comfortable as possible. She had a marvelous six weeks and then died at home.

For an elderly patient who is frail and weak, the intensive chemotherapy required to treat the acute leukemia of this patient simply caused excessive discomfort without any positive results. Treatment could easily cost between $20,000 to $50,000 with all of the likely hospitalization for complications, to say nothing of the tremendous physical and emotional costs.

The issue of terminal care is frequently encountered in caring for cancer patients. The physician must determine at the outset if the care is to be of a curative or palliative nature. He or she must be continually mindful of the purpose of treatment while managing the patient's care. The physician must also be willing to recognize that the purpose of treatment may change at some point, and be ready to alter their plans for the patient's care.

In determining what type of care to provide, one must consider the medical consequences of that treatment, as well as the social and financial consequences. There are substantial numbers of patients who undergo chemotherapy and/or radiation and suffer a high level of side effects without appreciable benefit. There are also those patients who may initially appear hopeless who after treatment show great improvement in their quality of life and longevity. It takes a considerable amount of experience, and at times, luck, to identify which of those borderline patients would likely benefit from treatment. Doctors need to talk with patients and their families before any treatment is begun and agree upon the strategies and alternatives. When patients are critically ill, treatment costs overall are very high. Families can easily wipe out years of savings for a few added weeks of survival. Experts in the field should establish guidelines that define appropriate care for specific tumor types. Physicians could use these to make determinations. The guidelines would have to be updated regularly to reflect changes in current treatments available in order to be of real clinical value.

Our system makes generous payments for terminal care but not for routine mammography for breast or sigmoidoscopy for colon cancer detection. We allow the bulk of our resources to be spent on hopeless, irreversible situations when coverage for early detection and prevention techniques could be more beneficial and less costly, according to Dr. Dan Deutschman, former president of the Cleveland Academy of Medicine.

Preventive Care

Blood pressure control, fitness and weight reduction counseling and anti-smoking programs could save untold medical dollars. By helping people control and correct these problems *before* they become severely ill, we can substantially reduce costly preventable diseases and their treatments.

In some situations, however, preventive care screening can be classified as inappropriate care. While preventive care has its value in terms of early detection and better treatment results in some areas, it is not always cost-effective. The cost of mass screening and follow-up are often greater than the savings realized from early detection. The frequency of mammography screening for women has recently been the subject of debate. We should re-examine the current recommendation that women over the age of 50 have annual mammograms. Since approximately one out of 10 women will develop breast cancer during their entire life, if we start doing yearly mammograms after age 50, we are doing a mammogram on 90 percent of women who will never have cancer of the breast. It would be wise, therefore, to do a study to determine who needs mammograms yearly, or every three years, or every five years. That is, determine who is most at risk to develop breast cancer and follow these patients more closely. Because of the explosion in lawsuits for failure to detect breast cancer early, a significant number of women are now having mammograms done two or three times annually because the radiologist is unsure or unwilling to commit himself when interpreting the mammogram. It is wrong to be satisfied with the recommendation that women after 50 should have a yearly mammogram when in some cases every five years may be adequate.

Equally important, is the fact that we should devise a more practical and sensible approach to dealing with women below 50, especially in the 30's and 40's. In my own practice, a significant number of breast cancer patients are in their mid 30's and mid 40's. It is not logical or cost-effective to do yearly mammograms on women 60 and over when about 85 percent will never develop breast cancer. And even in the cases where they do, it is usually less aggressive. Breast cancer in women between 30 and 40, unless discovered early, is often very aggressive and fatal. This is really the age group for whom we must develop a coherent and sensible screening program.

An MRI procedure which can cost about $1000 is now available to detect early breast cancer. However, in the current financial climate, institutions are unwilling to buy equipment costing $2 million. Some of the high-tech companies now admit that they have the capability to develop ultrasound machines which cost much less and provide very accurate diagnoses. We clearly need to develop a climate which encourages cost-effective screening methods rather than big ticket technologies and establish better standards of preventive care guidelines.

Cholesterol screening of all adults has been recommended by several medical organizations and government offices. The sudden surge in cholesterol screening centers in drug stores, shopping malls and free-standing clinics is not intended to provide factual data on which treatment will be based. This test is intended for screening purposes only and any physician would repeat the test under more controlled and precise circumstances before making any recommendations for treatment.

The cost of staffing and operating these programs, as well as the cost of arranging the necessary follow-up care for all patients with abnormal screening tests could be better spent on providing some basic care services to those without any care. Furthermore, cholesterol screening can be easily and efficiently incorporated into a patient's routine physical exam with their family doctor. Simply because we have the technology to perform an on-the-spot cholesterol screen in shopping malls, doesn't mean it is the most effective use of resources.

The Peer Review Board

There have been various attempts to change the behavior of physicians by setting up peer reviews or other monitoring systems. They have not worked due to faulty design. These review boards have been unsuccessful at tackling the problem and, in many instances, have actually added to the excessive costs of medical care. In discussing this problem with my colleagues, many agree that it makes no sense to allow doctors to perform procedures of questionable value and then try to review the circumstances of the procedure afterward.

Instead, we propose that a monitoring system be set up in each hospital to intervene and prevent excessive or unnecessary procedures before treatment is rendered. Rather than have a group of monitoring physicians meet monthly to review 50 to 100 charts, as is the current practice, it would be far more effective for each hospital to have a board comprised of two or three highly-trained doctors—not dependent on other doctors for referrals or income—and several skilled nurses to concurrently review selected patients' progress in the hospital. This panel could advise physicians and discourage questionable procedures. These doctors must be given sufficient authority to carefully monitor performance without interfering with the care of patients. They should focus on problem areas so that corrective or preventive actions could be recommended before they occur. This process would significantly reduce unnecessary procedures and care. The salary of these doctors and nurses would be paid from a pool funded by the hospitals, commercial insurers and Medicare. They would work on behalf of all parties to reduce costs and protect patients. They should also be protected from frivolous lawsuits. The physicians must be board- certified and well trained in the peer review process.

Currently most peer review is done after the fact and does not necessarily detect or stop waste. This process would be enormously beneficial to all those concerned with producing high quality care at an affordable price. Doctors would benefit because they would not receive daily calls from insurance companies to obtain progress reports and second-guess everything they do for hospitalized patients. Medicare would benefit because it currently spends a considerable amount of money on peer review. This process could be streamlined to achieve savings in their pre- and post-payment claims review systems. One large private insurance company maintains about 1,000 nurses and 50 doctors nationwide on its review panel. A peer review board on the local level would allow consolidation of peer review departments within insurance companies. This mechanism would go a long way toward curtailing unnecessary care without frustrating doctors. It would also lower the costs for hospitals, especially for cases in which they are paid a flat fee based on the diagnosis, regardless of the length of the patient's stay.

Under this plan, Medicare spending would also decrease because of the reduced number of services. It would be more equitable and fair to reduce excessive services than to continue to reduce the payment on services to a point that the hospitals and doctors are losing money taking care of Medicare patients. Further reductions in reimbursement by Medicare for needed and legitimate services might lead doctors to reject large numbers of Medicare patients because they cannot afford to care for these patients below cost.

Dr. Robert Brook of The Rand Corporation, one of the foremost authorities on health care issues and statistics, is a supporter of this concurrent review concept. It is imperative to realize, however, that in order to make this type of system work we must have a sound and equitable malpractice reform to allow people to do their work without fear of having unreasonable legal challenges every step of the way.

Development of Untapped Resources

Community health clinics must play a pivotal role in providing access to health care and controlling costs. The role for nurse practitioners, physician assistants and social workers should be expanded. Many of them should have additional training in specialized areas so they can provide expanded care in a competent manner under the supervision of a few doctors. Resident doctors who are specializing could be a source of help, in addition to a large number of retired doctors and nurses who would be happy to volunteer.

Rural health care has been a problem in that even insured patients have difficulty finding a doctor. This is why employing the concept of the community health clinic in rural areas would be vital. The December 13, 1993 issue of *Medical Economics* presents a very interesting way of attracting doctors to rural areas. It describes several highly trained doctors who needed a change in their student visa status in order to remain in the U.S. They were offered assistance in exchange for the opportunity to work in a rural area for two years. Most of them have stayed after their tour of duty. The same article suggested that Canadian family physicians could be a source of ample help to staff these areas since Canada has a surplus of family physicians and is trying desperately to curtail the number of doctors, particularly family physicians. This arrangement would only require a minimum change in immigration requirements since Canadian doctors do not have to take any special examination to work in the U.S.

Another important means of reducing health care costs is to develop cooperation between insurance companies, hospitals and physicians. At times these working relationships are not harmonious; however, all sides realize the necessity of give and take to be able to survive. There are two models we can observe that have accomplished managed competition in a free market without government intervention—1) The Rochester Plan and 2) The Cleveland Experience. Both plans rely heavily on pressuring hospitals and doctors to become more economical.

The Rochester Plan demonstrated significant reduction in health care costs through free market competition. While this plan depends on negotiation with hospitals and doctors, about 50 percent of the Rochester population is enrolled in an HMO. Premiums are community-rated, meaning that everybody in Rochester pays the same price for coverage. With nationwide premium costs now averaging $3600 per employee, the Rochester rate is $2400, a 30 percent rate reduction. The average hospital cost in Rochester is $400 per day versus $600 nationally. Rochester insurance administration costs are also about one-half the national average at six percent. Furthermore, only six percent of the people living in Rochester are uninsured.

Cleveland has also distinguished itself by making strides to control costs. In 1987, with double digit medical inflation raging all over the country, Ohio passed the Health Insurance Reform Act which permitted Blue Cross and Blue Shield of Ohio to negotiate selectively with hospitals to reduce prices. In the early 1980's, Cleveland was experiencing 16 percent annual inflation in the cost of an average hospital stay and ranked as the fourth most expensive city in the nation for hospital costs. But in 1990, the national hospital inflation rate was approximately eight percent while Cleveland held inflation to only 1.6 percent. In 1991, Cleveland hospitals' inflation rate of four percent was still about half the national average of 8.3 percent and Cleveland ranked 19th nationwide in hospital costs—a significant improvement.

Between 1985 and 1991 Blue Cross and Blue Shield of Ohio kept the increase in policy cost to about five percent, while the national average was about 13 percent. Also of note is that Cleveland has 10 percent uninsured compared to 14 to 16 percent nationwide. Ohio, as a matter of fact, measures 40th in the nation in the incidence of uninsured. No doubt job creation or relative availability of jobs has much to do with the reduced number of uninsured people.

This led John Burry, Jr., Chairman and CEO of Blue Cross and Blue Shield of Ohio to conclude that "before we seriously consider raising taxes and rationing care, I suggest we cut spending and reduce waste first...Yes, there is more than enough money right now to take care of the health care needs of every American. But it is also the duty of Americans to become prudent users of health care if this is going to work." Mr. Burry's analysis of health care costs may be found in the Summer 1993 issue of Blue Cross and Blue Shield of Ohio and Blue Shield, Summer of 1993, Vol. 1, Issue 2.

Obviously these plans are still under constant cost pressure. If only a few of the cost saving measures presented in this book were implemented, the Cleveland and Rochester plans could be even more affordable. For example, when a Rochester physician was informed that he was doing too many unnecessary procedures, he at first did not like the admonition. However, he did re-evaluate and change his practice pattern.

It would be pointless to call for change in physician's practice patterns, however, and not recognize the enormous need for simultaneous judicial reform. The medical community is acutely aware that medical costs will never come down until the liability epidemic is under control. The fear of litigation influences virtually every medical decision we make—from scheduling an appointment, prescribing a drug, or making a referral, to ordering a hospital admission, performing major surgery, or withdrawing life-support.

With the necessary reforms to our malpractice system, we can remove the incentive to perform unnecessary procedures as a means of self-preservation. By utilizing an on-site panel to review procedures *before* they are performed, we can help physicians make the most well-informed decisions about their patients' care and treatment. Without changes in these two key areas, we will never break the cycle of malpractice-driven unnecessary and inappropriate care.

CHAPTER 4

A Call for Medical Malpractice Reform: The Role Lawyers Play

In principle, the purpose of medical malpractice litigation is to fairly compensate injured patients and punish the negligent or incompetent professional. In practice, the United States' medical tort system does neither. Dr. Kathleen Weaver, M.D. notes that victims receive only 20 to 30 percent of all the premium dollars paid by physicians and hospitals (*Internist,* October; 1991). Ironically, suits are filed in only a small percentage of cases where the physician was, in fact, negligent. Furthermore, more than half of each damage award dollar goes to lawyer's fees and expenses. It seems the justifiably harmed are not being compensated for their injuries. Dr. Weaver expresses the outrageousness of this situation when she asks if any other segment of our economy would tolerate such high overhead and waste. Punishment for negligence is delivered in the form of monetary awards to victims. However, award money comes from insurance companies who pass the cost on to *all* physicians, not just those who are negligent. In turn, the physician passes the cost of rising malpractice insurance premiums on to the consumer.

Any effort to contain health care costs or reform the prevailing delivery system must take into account the effect malpractice suits are having on the U.S. economy. Each year the U.S. spends an estimated $300 billion as an indirect cost of the civil justice system. This problem is most acute in the medical field but it also impacts other markets. The cost of doing business in the United States, in terms of product liability, is 15 to 20 times higher than in Europe or Japan according to a report from former President Bush's Council on Competitiveness. U.S. physicians are 10 times more likely to be sued for malpractice than Canadian physicians. The cost of malpractice insurance is, correspondingly, 8 to 10 times higher than in Canada.

Does this imply that U.S. goods and products are 20 times inferior to Japanese and European goods? Or that our doctors are 10 times more incompetent than Canadian doctors? Perhaps the answer lies in the disproportionate number of lawyers practicing in the U.S. While the U.S. accounts for *only five percent* of the world's population, *we have 70 percent* of the world's lawyers. This translates into one lawyer for every 250 people. On the other hand, in Japan, there is one lawyer for every 10,000 people. Washington, D.C., the most litigious city in the country, has at least one lawyer for every ten people.

The abuse and overuse of the medico-legal system in this country is creating an enormous economic handicap. We cannot continue to compete in the world market with our current system of civil law. Efforts to bring about medical malpractice reform have been met with opposition. One argument is that restricting the number of suits filed or the size of available awards, denies victims the opportunity to seek compensation for their injuries. The call for malpractice reform, however, is by no means an initiative to eliminate meritorious cases. Rather, it is a desire for truth, justice and fair compensation for all victims, and speedy relief for those who are falsely accused!

Lawyers and Doctors at Odds

A Harvard study analyzing medical injury and malpractice in New York state, found that while three percent of medical treatments had bad results, negligence was evident only one percent of the time. Furthermore, the study found that there was no lawsuit filed in most of the cases in which negligence was evident. Thus, it seems that the number of lawsuits filed has little to do with negligence or adverse results. Why then are American doctors under the knife? What makes an attorney file suit and vigorously pursue a case that has no merit?

It would help, perhaps, to understand that lawyers are trained to represent the interests of their clients—truth and justice are of little importance to the majority of lawyers. The primary objective is to win! And, of course, there is the enticement of money. Litigation of a mere 40 cerebral palsy cases with a 50 percent success rate, could net a small law firm $50 million.

It was financial gain that led one former New York lawyer to sell cerebral palsy cases to other New York law firms. Employees at the rehabilitation centers where the patients resided, sold the confidential records to the lawyer for $2,000 per record. The lawyer would then sell the information to various law firms who would contact the patient's family and solicit them to file suit. The lawyer confessed to the grand jury that he had earned $1.5 million selling these confidential patient files.

Most medical malpractice suits have little or nothing to do with negligence. The major reason patients and lawyers are litigious is usually due to some major bodily harm—as in the case of cerebral palsy. Peter Huber, former law clerk to Supreme Court Justice, Sandra Day O'Connor, discusses the issue of cerebral palsy malpractice cases and vividly illustrates my point. He stated that annually, 4,000 children born in the U.S. develop cerebral palsy. Ten percent of all natural births are regarded as difficult deliveries, which is considered to be a possible cause of cerebral palsy. However, each year about 400 cerebral palsy cases with delivery difficulties end up in litigation. Expert witnesses assert that the difficult delivery was, in fact, the cause of the cerebral palsy and that better use of fetal monitoring and early caesarian section could have prevented the result. The jury sees the helpless child in a wheelchair and, feeling sorry for the family, gives a huge award.

Though electronic fetal monitoring is imprecise as an indicator of fetal distress, it has nonetheless, fueled a great many malpractice claims by providing a paper record of a "clear indication of fetal problems" to which the obstetrician failed to respond appropriately. Consequently, the number of caesarian births in the U.S. has risen from five percent in 1970 to about 25 percent in 1993. The cost of a caesarian birth is twice the cost of a normal vaginal delivery.

A few unscrupulous lawyers are abusing the legal system and milking the health care system. Many of the cases they file are without merit, simply causing further delays and backlogs in the courts. Dr. Donavin Baumgartner, M.D., Jr., contributing editor to *Cleveland Physician*, cites a few examples of frivolous lawsuits.

- A surgeon was sued for a negligent vasectomy when the patient's wife became pregnant. Even when independent testing proved the man's semen did not carry any sperm, the suit was not dropped.
- Another suit was filed against a doctor for not making the correct diagnosis and not requesting a consultation with a specialist. The hospital chart clearly showed that the consultation was requested and that the child's mother signed the child out of the hospital against medical advice before the consultant arrived.

Attorneys frequently name all doctors mentioned in a chart without investigating whether they had any involvement in the problem. A radiologist was sued for correctly reading a patient's chest x-ray. The patient required an appendectomy and suffered complications. The chest x-ray had no bearing on the case, however, the radiologist had to defend himself incurring expense, anxiety and loss of time from other worthwhile pursuits. An over zealous attorney named a Dr. Klspp as at fault in a case, not realizing this was an abbreviation for a group practice mentioned in the chart, not an individual physician.

Medical Expert Witness: Alias Hired Gun

Attorneys are not the only ones doctors fear when it comes to professional liability. There are an increasing number of physicians serving as expert witnesses who are more than willing to find malpractice in any cases presented to them. The proliferation of lawsuits and their profitability have spawned a new type of medico-legal consulting firm. Supplying "expert witnesses" has become big business. Consulting firms make adamant claims that their expert witnesses are not *professional* witnesses. Whether medical expert witnesses are testifying for a consulting firm or not, a doctor who makes a career of testifying against his or her medical colleagues solely for income deserves the alias, "hired gun."

We swear in court to tell the truth, the whole truth and nothing but the truth. But since the early 1970's the courts have essentially done away with this moral decree. Up until that point, testimony by an expert witness would only be admitted if it had gained general acceptance in the particular field. Here are several examples of hired guns caught lying.

A general surgeon, who specialized for many years in emergency medicine, offered his services as an expert witness for the plaintiff. He testified that he was board certified in thoracic surgery and professed to be a Phi Beta Kappa graduate from Williams College in 1959. In fact, he graduated from Ohio State in 1957. He also claimed that he graduated first in his class and was a member of Alpha Omega Alpha. However, it was discovered that he was not first in his class nor was he ever a member of the honor society.

In another incident, an orthopedic surgeon testified that he was board certified, when in fact, he had failed the board three times. When confronted on the witness stand, he stuck to his story, even though the judge warned him that he could be charged with perjury. After the Executive Director of the Board of Orthopedic Surgery flew in to testify that indeed the surgeon had failed the board three times, the orthopedic surgeon admitted that he was lying.

Another expert witness testified that he was affiliated with a major teaching hospital. Under cross-examination he was confronted with a cease and desist order from the hospital with which he claimed to be affiliated. It was brought out in court that he had long ago lost his practice privileges at the hospital for dishonorable reasons.

In an article published in *Medical Economics*, May 23, 1994, Dr. Robert J. Lerer, a developmental pediatrician in Cincinnati with extensive experience in medical malpractice work, states that it is not just plaintiffs' experts who fudge the truth. He says both sides are guilty and proposes reforms to stop the distortions.

He gave an example of a *plaintiff's* expert witness who is a distinguished professor who worked exclusively in the laboratory examining brain tissues claiming that he routinely worked in the intensive care unit taking care of children. On cross-examination, it was obvious he knew very little about clinical medicine. Even one of his former students testified that the professor had no direct patient care experience.

Dr. Lerer also complained of tailored testimony for the plaintiff. Such a case involved a girl who developed severe mental retardation starting at age four months. The obstetrician was sued for not performing a C-section. The plaintiff's attorney found a well-known expert witness to state that oxygen deprivation at birth was responsible for the mental retardation. This same expert had testified and written several times for the defense stating that, in fact, such neurological damage is never possible under similar circumstances. This contradictory testimony was so glaring that the jury ruled in favor of the defense.

Dr. Lerer cites several examples in which the *defense* expert witness was obviously lying. In one instance, the defense star witness was a distinguished M.D./Ph.D. from a university hospital. This witness invented a disease he called a "rare syndrome involving complex metabolic pathways in the liver" to explain the child's brain damage. Fortunately, the jury did not buy this.

Another neurologist was caught clearly contradicting himself. Dr. Lerer stated that the neurologist's testimony was so illogical that the expert witness was caught in his own distortions. A child's brain damage was due to meningitis, but the neurologist claimed that much brain damage could only be caused by genetic abnormalities. It was pointed out to him his own earlier articles contradicted his testimony. The jury did not believe him either.

Another *defense* expert, a well-known geneticist testified that a child's abnormal genes were responsible for his brain damage. In fact, all the evidence supported oxygen deprivation as the culprit and showed the child's chromosomes were perfectly normal. Dr. Lerer commented that he was not sure whether the geneticist was deliberately lying, but he did not expect such poor performance from such an authority.

While there are a lot of excellent physicians who testify on both sides, the system is fraught with corrupt and unsuccessful doctors who are determined to crucify their fellow physicians for pay. They often get away with it because there is no standard of competency established for these people who call themselves an expert witness and nobody prosecutes them for lying. Clearly the system needs changing.

Dr. Lerer said he could only speculate that the experts distort the truth due to greed and, at times, conceit. He suggests that when an expert is caught seriously distorting the truth, he or she should be permanently banned from ever testifying again. He also suggests each side should have more than one expert witness because blatant distortions are most common when one side has only one expert. He concluded that fortunately, despite the impression he may have given in his article, most expert witnesses in fact are quite honest and competent.

Dr. Charles C. Norland, M.D. of Missouri Baptist Medical Center, presents an insightful analysis of the effects of our present legal system on the practice of medicine in his article "Liability Epidemic" (*Missouri Medicine,* April 1992). He calls attention to two prominent authors on the liability issue, Peter Huber, currently a Senior Fellow at the Manhattan Institute and Walter Olson, former president of the American Bar Association.

Huber states in an article entitled "Junk Science in the Courtroom," (*Forbes,* July 8, 1991) that "an expert who appears in court to present nothing but his own idiosyncratic opinions is, for all practical purposes, just a lawyer in scientific drag. Science, by definition, is never a matter of individual opinions; it is always a matter of consensus in a much larger community."

Olson, author of *The Litigation Explosion,* writes that a federal judge once commented that "an expert witness can be found to testify to the truth on any factual matter, no matter how frivolous." In his analysis of the relationship of our legal system and medical practice, Dr. Norland concludes that when we allow "junk scientists" to take control of the court system, physicians are forced to live and practice in fear. Furthermore, when physicians fear being sued for each move they make, they have no other choice but to practice "defensive" medicine at great cost to us all.

High Cost of Defensive Medicine

America is in the grips of a malpractice epidemic. This crisis began in the 1970's and peaked in the latter half of the 1980's. The Insurance Information Institute reports that the number of malpractice claims dropped from a peak in 1985, but the number of claims seeking more than $1 million has increased steadily. In 1988, the number of $1 million claims was up 25 percent over 1987. In the first four months of 1989, the number of claims had already exceeded the 1988 total.

At least 15 percent of the total cost of physician services are related to medical malpractice, i.e., the cost of insurance premiums and defensive medicine, according to information from the Insurance Information Institute, January 1991. In a survey, doctors were asked to name the 12 principal causes of increasing health care costs. Malpractice litigation was rated number one by 93 percent of those surveyed. Other causes ranking high on the list were administrative costs for insurance, drug costs, patient demand, inappropriate or unnecessary care and doctors' fees. The American public is generally unaware of the frequency at which doctors are sued for malpractice. Many of these cases are settled out of court because the physician, understandably, wants to avoid a visible trial—even in those cases where they are certain they have not been negligent.

Various estimates put the total malpractice premium and related expense for U.S. doctors at $25 billion with another $21 billion spent on defensive medicine. Other experts, including former U.S. Surgeon General, C. Everett Koop, believe the cost of defensive medicine is near $63 billion. While it is very difficult to arrive at a precise cost of defensive medicine, the medical community knows that far too many services are performed out of a perceived need to pursue all possible diagnoses, no matter how unlikely, as protection in the event of a lawsuit.

A recent survey by the American Medical Association found that 70 percent of doctors ordered excessive numbers of consultations with specialists and nearly the same number ordered more tests than were necessary, to guard against liability claims. Practicing defensive medicine doesn't really safeguard doctors from lawsuits, it merely provides the illusion of protection. In a report published in October, 1991, in the *Journal of the American Medical Association*, 1400 cases involving lawsuits were reviewed. Of those 1400, less than 15 percent were associated with failure to order diagnostic tests.

Consider an example of a diabetic patient admitted to the hospital by his internist for treatment of biliary colic. Laboratory results showed that the patient was slightly anemic. The patient was then referred to a hematologist prior to the surgery for evaluation of the anemia. The endocrinologist was brought in for management of the diabetes and a cardiologist evaluated the patient to give pre-operative cardiac clearance. Each of these specialists submitted a bill for consultation, ordered some tests and possibly some follow-up after the patient's discharge. Unless the situation was unusually complicated, the internist was capable of handling this case alone.

Performing more tests and referring patients to specialists often serves only to reinforce the patient's notion that their condition is more serious than it may be, and that the doctor is unable to find a cause or solution. This is particularly true in cases with vague symptoms for which a cause is often never found.

Until there is significant change in our tort system, already scarce health dollars will continue to be wasted on defensive medical practices. Alfred A. de Lorimier, President of the American Pediatric Surgical Association, writes in the *Journal of Pediatric Surgery*, March 1993, that one-third of the cost of a pint of blood is the cost of liability insurance. Similarly, *95 percent* of the cost of childhood vaccines is due to liability insurance costs for the pharmaceutical manufacturer and the physician. On May 17, 1994, Ohio Governor George Voinovich expressed his frustration that most of the cost of vaccination is due to exorbitant liability premiums and that a meaningful malpractice reform is desperately needed. Every $100 the patient pays to the doctor includes $11 for malpractice insurance. To break it down further: $50 goes to pay for the doctor's overhead and 40 to 50 percent of the remainder goes to pay for taxes, leaving about $25. If less than one percent of patients seen by doctors develop treatment injuries, why do we spend as much as 50 percent of doctors' take home revenue to cover malpractice awards?

Emotional Toll on Doctors

Much attention has been focused on the actual dollar cost of malpractice insurance as a contributing factor to the overall health care crisis. Very little attention is paid to the actual physical, emotional, psychological and spiritual costs to physicians and health care professionals as a result of unnecessary lawsuits. In most instances, the cases are dismissed, but the damage has already been done by the mere filing of these frivolous suits. These cases create a considerable amount of stress on the physician. Few people can relate to the anguish, anger and fear that go along with a malpractice suit filed against a doctor.

"From the first days of medical education, we put the fear of lawsuits above the fear of God, into our young doctors," states Dr. Sidney Sharzer, a California obstetrician who has extensive experience in medical malpractice cases (*Medical Economics*, March 1993). "In some magical way," he continues, "they [doctors] think that covering every possibility, no matter how remote or what the cost, will absolve them from responsibility for bad results. They tend to forget that bad results happen no matter what you do."

Many doctors are quitting high risk specialty practices because of the increasing likelihood of being sued. As a result, access to care is being seriously impaired, especially in some rural and semi-rural areas. Certain high-risk specialty care is unavailable to the residents of these small towns, whether they have insurance or not.

Malpractice suits have also played a major role in the destruction of the once familial doctor-patient relationship. One California doctor related his experience of being sued six times in his 20 years of general practice in an article in *Medical Economics,* March 1992. He says each suit had a profound effect on the way he practiced medicine and he admitted that he has become cynical, suspicious and is no longer fascinated with the practice of medicine. The following cases involving this doctor are typical of the kind of frivolous and destructive lawsuits brought against physicians practicing in the United States.

The first case involved a patient who became dizzy while having his blood drawn in the doctor's office. He was put in bed but got up on his own and fainted. He suffered no injuries from the fall and was put back in bed. They watched him and gave him cookies and juice. The patient was fine after several hours and went home with no subsequent problems. However, three years later he sued the doctor for letting him get out of bed too early. The trial lasted three days with the jury finally deciding in favor of the doctor.

The second case involved a lady admitted to the hospital for pneumonia. After a slow recovery she was finally scheduled to be discharged. Shortly before her discharge the patient's blood pressure dropped abruptly. She collapsed and died. Being well acquainted with the family, the doctor spent a considerable amount of time consoling them. However, three days before the statute of limitations expired he received notice of lawsuit. After many hours of conferences and depositions, the plaintiff's own expert witness completely cleared the doctor of any wrong-doing. The conclusion was that the woman probably died of a heart attack.

This same doctor had another patient who never complied with his recommendations. The patient had chronic multiple complaints and underwent several coronary artery studies which were all negative. One day he suffered a puncture wound and was treated. He was asked to come back for follow up, but never did. Later the patient developed osteomyelitis, an infection of the bone. He sued the doctor. After several hours of depositions the plaintiff's lawyer decided to drop the case because he could not find an expert witness to claim that the patient's care was below the normal standard.

Another case involved a young man who drank heavily, abused drugs and frequently beat his wife. One day the man slammed his fist through the window of his front door. He sought medical treatment; later suing the doctor for not finding the retracted tendon. Despite the fact that all the expert witnesses advised his lawyer the tendon actually could not have been repaired, the lawyer prepared his case for trial anyway. His thinking was that a jury would feel sorry for his client because he had subsequently become paralyzed after an automobile accident. This case was dismissed by the judge as unworthy. The doctor lost several days of office appointments with patients and countless nights of sleep. His anxiety was, in his words, "close to overwhelming."

The doctor was again sued for the death of a patient following surgery for a ruptured spleen. The anesthesiologist involved in this case settled out of court. The doctor also settled out of court upon the advice of his insurance company lawyer. In spite of the small settlement, every time he fills out an application he has to state that he has settled a case out of court.

Another suit filed against the doctor involved a 19-year-old boy who suffered minor injuries when his motorcycle crashed into a dirt bank. He was treated in the emergency room for facial abrasions and contusions and sent home. When the boy came back later for treatment of his wounds, he was running a low grade fever and was started on antibiotics.

Two days later, the patient reported that his temperature was back to normal and that he was not experiencing any nausea or headaches. However, he did complain of having a stiff back and neck, which he attributed to the accident. The doctor prescribed an anti-inflammatory medication to ease the pain and stiffness in his neck and back. When the boy's parents left for work the next day, the boy assured them he was feeling better. When the family returned home later that evening, they found him comatose. He was diagnosed with meningitis and died two days later without ever regaining consciousness.

The patient's CAT scan and facial x-rays were negative but an autopsy found a minute fracture of the cribriform plate which probably was the source of the cerebrospinal fluid contamination. The boy's family subsequently filed a malpractice suit against the doctor, accusing him of negligence.

The doctor strongly disputed their claim and was ready to fight it out in court, armed with an array of experts, including an infectious disease specialist, a neurosurgeon, an internist and a neurologist. However, he decided to settle the case for $1 less than California's $30,000 floor for settlement amounts that must be reported to the licensing board. The doctor settled because he feared that if he held out and lost the case it would be a blemish on his record and his medical practice would be adversely affected.

When discussing with his colleagues the malpractice cases brought against him, the doctor discovered that many of them had similar stories to tell. *Medical Economics*, December 1992, reports a malpractice ordeal of a family practitioner in Michigan. She concluded that even a person with the most notorious criminal offense has a constitutional right for a speedy trial, but she asserts those same privileges were not extended to her. When she was sued in 1979, her attorney advised her to prepare for the case to last two to three years. Ten years later, she finally pushed the case to a close after her crazed outburst about further trial delays.

The doctor said that she put an IUD in a patient without complication and gave her the usual instructions. She told the patient to come back for a check-up the next month, but the patient did not return until three months later when she was having pelvic pain. The IUD was removed and the examination and the lab culture showed the patient had gonorrhea. She was called and told to return immediately for antibiotics. She never came. After repeated calls, the patient finally appeared two months later. She continued to have pain after the antibiotic treatment and was referred to a gynecologist but never kept the appointment. Nearly two years later, the patient returned. During that time she had seen about 12 different doctors. Pelvic infection and tubal pregnancy had resulted in surgical removal of her fallopian tubes.

In 1979, this patient sued the doctor and the IUD manufacturer. The doctor learned that the patient did not want to sue her but the attorney pushed for the suit because he wanted to keep the case in the Michigan Circuit Court system. The case would have had to go to the U.S. District Court since the IUD manufacturer was out of state, unless the doctor was implicated.

A mediation panel, consisting of three trial attorneys, recommended a $50,000 award to the plaintiff to be paid by the IUD manufacturer. The doctor was found completely innocent. The patient and the doctor agreed to the settlement, but the IUD maker refused to accept the mediation recommendation. Subsequently, the manufacturer did everything possible to stonewall the proceedings. The judge refused to dismiss the case against the doctor and gave limitless extensions.

After 10 years a trial date was set. The doctor canceled all her office appointments for the entire week so she could resolve the case. Her lawyer made one last effort to convince the judge to have the claim against her dismissed, but the judge refused. Soon after, she learned that there was a similar case in the Michigan Appeals Court and both lawyers wanted to wait for the outcome of that appeal before continuing her case. She was told the appeal might last another two years.

At that point she became in her words, "maniacal". She informed her attorney that she was going to trial on the scheduled date whether there was one or not. The next step was to go to the Attorney General's office, then the Detroit Free Press and finally, to the Supreme Court and to park herself there until her case was heard. The attorney could see her determination and anger and went to plead with the judge. Since there was no material evidence, the judge finally agreed. Within 24 hours the case against her was dismissed.

For many doctors the fun and joy of practicing medicine has all but gone. They view patients as potential litigants, constantly worrying about being named in a frivolous lawsuit. Lawyers say that it is just business and should not be taken personally, but physicians *do* take it personally.

"Doctor Perfect"

Public perception in the U.S. is that all cases *can* and *should* be correctly diagnosed—regardless of the type and manner of symptoms exhibited. This is unreasonable and virtually impossible even with all the highly advanced technology available. Approximately eight percent of heart attack victims do not exhibit symptoms in such a way as to be identifiable when first seen. In children under the age of two, appendicitis is extremely difficult to diagnose. It is simply not a likely diagnosis because it rarely occurs in this age group.

Striving to live up to the public's expectations and not get sued in the process, forces doctors to practice defensive medicine, which significantly adds to the nation's health care bill. However, ordering more tests doesn't save physicians from malpractice and often proves unnecessary.

In *Medical Economics*, March 1993, a California obstetrician related his experience. A 14-week pregnant woman was involved in an auto accident. The seat belt had bruised her upper abdomen and chest—far away from her uterus. However, the obstetrical resident in the emergency room ordered a pelvic ultrasound and a detailed coagulation work-up. He wanted to admit the patient and repeat the coagulation work-up every twelve hours. But the patient felt fine and refused admission. She went home to be with her other child and subsequently had a normal delivery. The resident's response may have been an overreaction, but it illustrates the degree to which doctors fear lawsuits.

Malpractice Crisis Alive and Well

There are those who argue that there is no malpractice crisis or that the problem is abating. An article by Mark Crane in *Medical Economics*, October 24, 1994 clearly shows that the problem is alive and, in many ways, is much worse. It is a potentially disastrous situation. Crane, Senior Editor of *Medical Economics*, pointed out that primary care doctors are being sued more than ever. The result is steep increases in malpractice premiums which are now rising even faster than those of specialists.

Much of this increased legal action against primary care doctors can be attributed to managed care. Primary care doctors who are assigned to a "gate-keeper" role by the insurance company are being sued for failure to refer the patient to a specialist in a timely manner or failure to perform certain tests when the patient's outcome is not as expected. In other words, the insurance company says, in order to keep costs down, don't perform too many tests and don't be too quick to refer the patient to an expensive specialist. If the physician does not keep costs down for the insurance company, he or she can be dropped from the preferred provider list. But if the patient feels more testing should have been done or a specialist should have been consulted sooner, a lawsuit may follow.

Malpractice premiums vary widely all over the country depending on how litigious the locality is. In metropolitan Detroit, Michigan, the annual premium for a practicing obstetrician is $141,150. In parts of Florida and Texas, physicians in high risk specialties— obstetrics and neurosurgery—pay more than $100,000 a year in premiums. Typically, downstate New York pays two to three times higher premiums than upstate or rural New York. The following chart highlights some of the disparities.

	Internist	Surgeon	Obstetrician
New York			
Upstate	$ 9,000	$ 22,300	$ 43,000
Downstate	26,000	66,000	127,000
California	5–8,000	18–27,000	32–49,000
Florida	9–20,000	32–66,000	63–132,000
Michigan	14–25,000	41–78,000	68–141,000
Nevada	9–14,000	28–49,000	45–82,000
Ohio	6–10,000	22–33,000	34–52,000
Texas	5–19,000	18–112,000	37–134,000

Source: *Medical Liability Monitor, Medical Economics,* 10/24/94.

It is quite likely that the malpractice climate is worse than it appears. Doctors pay over $5 billion in insurance premiums each year. In spite of an uncertain malpractice climate, more and more malpractice insurers are springing up. A few years ago, everyone was avoiding the malpractice insurance business. Because of the host of recent earthquakes, tornadoes and floods with devastating consequences, the malpractice insurance business is becoming relatively appealing. Some experts predict that one more major earthquake or flood may put some of the property casualty insurance companies out of business.

Hence, there are many new insurers entering the malpractice insurance market. Many of these new companies will lose money and bail out. Many of the new competitors are using what Timothy Morse, vice-president of St. Paul Fire and Marine Insurance Health Care Professional division, calls predatory and irresponsible price-cutting to get business. Some premiums are as much as 40 percent below average. However, the number of claims is rising and the size of awards is greater. Since there is a lag time for claims to start appearing, it will take a few years for awards to catch up to these new companies. Many of the small, newly formed insurance companies will simply not have the resources to pay the awards when claims become due. It is, therefore, imperative that any malpractice reform address the issue that a number of fleeting insurance companies are collecting huge sums of premium dollars. These companies manage to never pay benefits and then disappear or declare bankruptcy when benefits are due.

Upon examining the chart above, the huge variation in premiums even within the individual states is apparent. Does this mean that the doctors in rural Michigan or Upstate New York are two to five times more competent and caring, and that they injure their patients less often than doctors in Detroit or Long Island?

In New York state, there was a 14 percent increase in premium in 1993 and another eight percent increase in 1994. Edward Amsler of Medical Liability Mutual Insurance company stated that the 19 percent increase was really the correct increase needed to meet expected claims and eight percent was merely a political decision which will eventually catch up with the politicians.

Obviously, most doctors in these high risk specialties simply cannot afford the $100,000 plus annual premium. As an alternative, doctors obtain coverage through hospitals or institutions by becoming employees of those facilities. Some doctors buy insurance coverage from potentially insolvent off-shore companies that may not deliver. Others simply have no coverage at all. When the doctor has no insurance and someone gets injured, who pays for it? The taxpayer pays. Amsler questioned how anyone can say we don't have a malpractice crisis when specialists are paying those kinds of premiums with no end in sight.

It is easy to put a large part of the blame on a "very active plaintiffs' bar" such as in Michigan. Lawyers on the whole are decent people who are struggling to meet the daily requirements of life and take care of their children and family like anyone else. What is at fault here is really the medico-legal system. We have created, over the years, a system that encourages abuse and predatory behaviors with absolute impunity. It is the medical malpractice system that urgently needs an overhaul.

Solutions for Ending the Malpractice Epidemic

Sound malpractice reform would accomplish at least one goal. It would provide adequate compensation for those who have been injured through medical practice. The solutions we propose are not radical or new. It is simply a matter of taking the best possible elements of different proposals and plans that are in existence and synthesizing them in a way that would protect both patients and physicians and be beneficial to lawyers. Obviously, there will be a few losers, namely, a handful of lawyers who are now abusing the system by filing frivolous lawsuits. By far the majority of lawyers are there to protect the interests of their clients. In addition, a small segment of physicians would also be affected, namely the ones who really have no business continuing the practice of medicine; those who are incompetent, usually the result of alcohol or drug abuse, and those who perpetually hurt patients and get away with it.

A starting point for tort reform can be found in the California system. In 1975, California decided to do something about escalating malpractice premiums. The legislature passed a law called the Medical Injury Compensation Reform Act (MICRA). Some claim that MICRA has reduced malpractice premiums by at least 25 to 30 percent. Howard Levine, President of Cleveland Academy of Medicine, feels that a nationwide plan like MICRA would further reduce premiums, partially because it reduces the likelihood of exposure to huge unrealistic malpractice awards.

Many plans with MICRA-like benefits are being considered in Congress right now. They have four major components:
1. Cap pain and suffering awards at $250,000.
2. Institute a sliding scale for attorney fees so the injured party gets a larger share of the award.
3. Spread awards over a period of time rather than a lump sum.
4. Notify the jury of other sources of compensation the victim has received.

Most of the serious proposals currently before Congress have included a cap of $250,000 on pain and suffering and some limitation on attorney fees, usually between 20 and 25 percent. Jim Cooper's bipartisan plan goes a little further and appears to be the most effective proposal to date. In addition to the $250,000 cap on pain and suffering, attorney fees are limited to 25 percent for the first $150,000 of the award and 10 percent of the remainder. However, it might be worthwhile to cap commission to the first million dollars so that anything above one million goes to the client. We must also set up a system that reduces costs for the attorney.

Once the client's award is made more equitable, the next stop is arbitration. A major problem with malpractice litigation is that it takes too long—at least two years to go to court and an average of five and a half years to resolve complicated cases. Some cases drag on for eight or 10 years. Alternative means of resolution, by mediation or arbitration, can help to reduce costs and shorten the length of conflict resolution. All malpractice cases should first go through arbitration unless both parties agree to proceed without it. The arbitration process must be simple, brief and inexpensive. The arbitrators must be people who are motivated to help resolve the malpractice dispute rather than people who are using their position to generate large sums of income or principally to supplement their income. They should also be certified in medical injury compensation issues. Many experts say that if arbitration is properly structured it will lead to faster resolution of cases, be less costly and produce less aggravation than a lawsuit.

However, arbitration can increase costs if the system gets bogged down. If the cases keep going to court, arbitration becomes inefficient. At the present time arbitration is either encouraged or required in about 50 percent of the states. In some areas, it works well. In others, it does not.

The Kaiser Permanente model of effective arbitration bears note. Kaiser Permanente, the largest HMO with over 2,000,000 members in northern California, requires members to agree to settle through arbitration any malpractice dispute that occurs during their care at Kaiser. Over 90 percent of these cases are resolved to the satisfaction of both parties and less than 10 percent of the cases go to court. Milton Cooper, Senior Legal Counsel for Kaiser Permanente, states that for the most part, both physician and patient are pleased with the arbitration. Grounds for appeal of the arbitration decision are limited to fraud, blatant prejudice or a refusal to hear evidence. Whenever an appeal is filed, the court will only vacate or affirm the award. If the award is affirmed, judgment is entered and must be paid.

The State of Maryland was one of the first to introduce arbitration. Walter R. Tabler, the chief health claim arbitrator, states that the system worked very well when first implemented in the 1970's, but has steadily broken down because of increasing case loads and people taking advantage of the system. One of the problems with the arbitration system, according to Tabler, is that "there is no way you can put teeth into the law" (*Impact*, February 1994).

Consequently, others like William Skinner, an attorney in Rockville, MD, observed that arbitration does not necessarily save money. In fact, it could be very expensive because you might end up paying up to $10,000 to three arbitrators and a court recorder and still end up in court and do it all over again. This is exactly what should not be allowed to happen. If arbitration is to be used effectively, it should not be voluntary. The law should be specific and not permit loopholes which make arbitration a charade. Furthermore, the "loser pays" rule must apply if people refute the verdict reached in arbitration and seek a court trial.

We must shift the emphasis of malpractice reform toward a humane goal—that is to adequately compensate people who have been injured during medical practice. It should not be a lottery for a handful of people to make a huge amount of money and leave uncompensated those who have been injured.

In order to simplify the process, we must have a pool of doctors who are competent and willing to evaluate and testify for both the plaintiff and the defendant. There is an abundance of competent people willing to do this. The names of these people should be made readily available. This would eliminate incompetent people who are unsuccessful in their medical practice and become the so-called "hired guns" who will say and do anything to make money. The expert witnesses should be required to take continuing medico-legal education courses and be certified.

Similarly the arbitration panel should be well versed in medico-legal issues and also be certified. We should devise ways to expedite the system and make it reasonably inexpensive for lawyers to be able to obtain certification that their cases are not frivolous. This has already been done in many states. Before legal counsel goes to arbitration or court, they have to prove that the case has merit by obtaining certification from at least two experts. Strict sanctions should be placed on lawyers who are guilty of repeatedly filing frivolous lawsuits. We must abolish once and for all the cruel system whereby you can sue all the doctors and personnel who cared for the patient whether or not they have anything to do with the alleged injury. It is the responsibility of the plaintiff's attorney to make a reasonable effort to identify the physician or physicians responsible for the injury. The defendant should be able to counter sue for injury if the plaintiff and/or his attorney know, or reasonably should know, that the case is without merit and refuse to withdraw it in a timely manner. Similarly, a referring physician should not be sued because he or she made a referral to a highly trained and well regarded specialist if an unavoidable bad result occurs. If, however, the referring physician sends a patient to a specialist who is well-known to have a problem or has a history of persistent bad results, then the referring physician may bear some responsibility for the bad result.

Also, there should be strict sanctions on doctors who deliberately lie about their credentials and expert witnesses who deliberately distort scientific facts for profit. The legal expert witnesses must be well recognized in the field in which they testify. They must be in active medical practice and be thoroughly familiar with current developments in their area of expertise. Punitive damages should be very carefully defined and the punishment should go to the appropriate person. If you have a physician who is impaired, refuses help, and continues to hurt patients, their license should be suspended until the doctor is no longer a menace to patients.

In summary, providing fair and reasonable compensation for victims of medical injury and giving a fair and reasonable share of that money to the legal counsel; having a mechanism to discipline incompetent doctors; providing abundant, honest and competent expert witnesses; and having a speedy arbitration or trial would save money and aggravation and significantly reduce the spiraling cost of health care. This, in turn, should lead to a significant reduction in malpractice premiums which will help to reduce the fees now charged for many high-priced procedures by at least 20 percent in some situations. Some of this revenue could then be shifted to family practitioners who, in many instances are inadequately compensated for the considerable amount of hours they spend in their practices.

Government may tinker all it wants with the current medical system, but until there is significant judicial reform, physicians will resist changes in health care delivery. From the many examples cited here, one can see that doctor's concerns are real, not imagined, and that many of the excessive procedures they perform are the result of excessive and unjustified medical malpractice lawsuits.

CHAPTER 5

A Look at Other Health Plans: What's Right for America?

America is not alone in her struggle against rising health care costs. Laurene Graig, a health care analyst at Wyatt Co., observed that "health care systems around the world are buckling under the pressure of aging population, exploding medical costs increases, and reliance on expensive high-tech solutions and procedures (*Investor's Business Daily*, April 1993). Britain's National Health Service, Canada's province-based systems, as well as the German and Japanese systems have received much attention from U.S. politicians and health care economists as possible models for U.S. health care reform. While we look elsewhere for answers, the fact is that most countries with government-run or nationalized health care systems are also struggling with spiraling cost increases. In varying degrees, they suffer from the same problems confronting the U.S. In some countries, the problems are compounded by highly restricted access and the depersonalization of care.

Health Care in Japan

The Japanese system provides health care at some of the lowest costs in the world. Total costs are about seven percent of GNP as opposed to America's nearly 13 percent. The financial load on businesses in Japan is only about one-fifth the burden borne by U.S. companies.

However, these remarkable achievements are not without a price. It is not unusual for patients in Japan to travel long distances and wait for six hours at a clinic for a very brief visit with the doctor. Visits are frequently made simply to dispense refills of prescribed medications. Since fees are strictly limited and the patient pays only about $7 a month for an unlimited number of doctor visits, selling prescription medications to their patients has become one of the primary income sources for Japanese doctors. It is no coincidence that the Japanese society is one of the world's largest consumers of prescription drugs.

The Japanese take at least 50 percent more drugs than Americans. Dr. Masanori Fukushima, a cancer specialist who has spent time working both in Japan and in the U.S., commented that a lot of these drugs are of dubious value since drug testing and efficacy are not strictly applied in Japan. Dr. Fukushima was quite impressed by the quality of the medical service provided in the U.S., and the close relationship that often develops between the doctor and patient—something that rarely exists in Japan.

Japanese doctors are not expected to give their patients much information about their treatment or condition. Labels are frequently removed from medications so patients do not even know what they are taking. James Sterngold of the New York Times cited an example of the patient's lack of information in an article printed in the December 28, 1992 issue. He told of a case in which the Japanese Supreme Court ruled that doctors need not inform patients that they have cancer. A woman refused surgery for what she had been told were gallstones and died. In reality, she had cancer but was not informed of that fact. Her family sued because they felt she would have made a different decision if she had known all the facts. The court, however, upheld the doctor's decision not to give the patient full information about her diagnosis. In addition, the Japanese system is beginning to grapple with some of the same issues that plague the U.S. system. The Japanese population over 65 is expected to double within thirty years, reaching 25 percent of the total population by 2020. According to data from the Japanese Ministry of Health and Welfare, costs for those over 65 are expected to increase from about

18 percent of health care spending in 1980 to 37 percent by 2000. Whereas the system was at one time generating a large surplus of funds which the insurance companies invested in resorts in Hawaii and Australia, insurance companies now recognize that large budget cuts and facility closings are inevitable. Japanese doctors are also worried about further controls on fees and the medications they prescribe.

While the Japanese system is currently facing some financial dilemmas, it has largely succeeded in keeping overall costs low. Only about half of the population is covered by corporate plans. Contrary to the U.S., Japanese businesses are not responsible for coverage of retirees since they are covered under a separate system. The average employee's cost for health care premiums is about three percent of their income and the amount is matched by the employer. The health ministry updates the national fee schedule, which determines the reimbursement to hospitals and physicians, every two years. Although patients may be responsible for 10 to 30 percent of the medical costs they incur, there are limits on the monthly liability. The system also provides subsidies to low income families.

Very importantly, there are other unique factors that have a significant impact on lower health care costs in Japan. First of all, the system is not suffering from the devastating effects of widespread poverty and violence that are seen in the U.S. The Japanese have a healthier diet than most Americans which also helps reduce demand on the system. Dr. Louis Sullivan observes that in spite of less medical sophistication, Japan excels in life expectancy and infant mortality. However, this is partially due to cultural reasons. He noted that we have more homicide in Washington, D.C. than the whole of Japan with a population of 130 million people. A 98 percent literacy rate, 99 percent of pregnant women receiving prenatal care and a diet low in fat content are also contributing factors in lower costs. Perhaps most notably, malpractice suits are rare and the legal system does not contribute to rising health care costs.

In spite of tight price controls, per capita health care spending in Japan has increased 145 percent in the ten-year period ending in 1991, according to data from the Organization of Economic Cooperation and Development. Besides prescription drug costs, hospital costs are a major factor in sharply rising health care costs.

The average hospital stay in Japan is almost 40 days, compared to an average of six days in the United States. The cost per day is relatively low which helps keep overall costs down. Low fees, however, may encourage doctors to keep the patient in the hospital longer to increase revenues. This is exactly what was happening in this country about 15 years ago when physicians were encouraged to keep as many patients in the hospital as long as possible and the hospitals made more money. At that time, Medicare and private insurance companies simply paid the bills when submitted. Now the Japanese system is facing the dire consequences of this approach.

The control of doctor's fees is extremely strict. The Japanese government decides what procedures will be covered and how much may be charged. There is no recognition of skill or expertise in the fee structure, nor are variations in the cost of providing the service in various regions of the country taken into account. An experienced specialist in a demanding field of medicine is paid the same for an examination as a new general practitioner. This approach encourages a focus on quantity of services provided since expertise, skill and the cost of providing a service are not recognized. This is alarmingly similar to the current trend in the Medicare fee schedule in the U.S. and the philosophies behind it.

Emikio Ohnuki-Tierney, a University of Wisconsin professor studying the Japanese health care system, observed two doctors in a private internal medicine clinic who, in the course of three hours, saw 100 outpatients for the first time and another 100 for repeat visits. During this same period, one doctor on duty at the eye clinic saw 48 patients. Another doctor at the ear, nose and throat clinic saw 45 patients. However, Japanese patients who can afford it often pay a "gratuity" in order to see the best specialists and avoid the long wait. This practice is simply recognized as being a part of the system.

The Japanese system is no miracle. After his visit to Japan, Dr. Louis Sullivan remarked that Japan spends much less on health care and it shows. He describes Japanese hospitals as a throw back to American hospitals of the 1950's—large hospital wards with four to eight patients per room, shared bathrooms located down the hall, and few modern facilities. He found that Japanese doctors see about 80 patients a day spending about three minutes per patient.

American doctors provide twice as much service for their patients. However, if one considers just the middle class in the U.S., the cost of providing care for U.S. citizens of similar health status to their Japanese counterparts may be the same or even less than the Japanese spend. This is due to the fact that 50 percent of healthy Americans consume only about three percent of all the health care dollars, as previously pointed out. So it is no miracle that Japan is able to provide "no frills" care for a homogeneous population, i.e., a similar well-educated middle class population. Americans, however, would likely reject the Japanese system's serious limitations and the impersonal nature of the doctor/patient relationship.

Health Care in Canada

There are many people who are fascinated with the Canadian system and want to have it adopted here in the U.S. However, the Canadian system would not work in the U.S. because Americans have very different values. Dr. Louis Sullivan agrees that there is "no silver bullet which some people want to believe in, such as the Canadian plan." The Canadian system has waiting lines which are often very long and amount to de facto rationing or deferral of services. Simply changing the system for collection of funds and distributing payments, although providing some potential reduction in paperwork, would not solve American health care problems because it would not address the unique problems that drive up health care costs in this country.

The fact that Canada, like all other industrialized countries, is having very serious budgetary problems demonstrates another reason the system is not suitable for the U.S. Canadians are actually looking at the U.S. system for guidance. An article by Clyde H. Farnsworth in the *New York Times*, March 7, 1993, entitled, "Now Patients are Paying Amid Canadian Cutbacks, Spending Outstrips Government's Ability to Pay," documents that Canadians are footing the bill even for routine lab work, like throat cultures. While patients bearing financial responsibility for their care is unheard of in the 27-year history of universal insurance in Canada, it is likely to become commonplace as the government finds itself increasingly unable to cover the costs of the nation's health care bill.

The Canadian medical system encourages doctors to provide unnecessary services. Estimates by Canadian health economists suggest that one-third of all elective surgery in Canada is unnecessary. And like Japan, prescription drug consumption is on the rise. These factors make health care the largest and most rapidly growing item in provincial budgets. At the current growth rates, within 10 years health care spending will make up nearly 50 percent of the budget of most provinces.

Goeffrey York, a guest editorialist in the *Journal of Public Health Policy*, Summer of 1992, pointed out that large numbers of Canadian patients regularly see physicians without real need, partly because of the country's fee structure. He tells of some doctors who run their offices like factories. One rural doctor in Manitoba was seeing about 80 to 90 patients a day. There is evidence that this type of practice style is becoming increasingly common in the Canadian health care system. Many doctors visits are made by patients who have no medical illness. According to York, these patients suffer from stress, anxiety, depression and other psychologically-oriented problems. When doctors treat these patients with merely a prescription, they return again and again for more medication which does not fix their problem. A former president of the Canadian Medical Association called the Canadian system "a monstrous and gigantic sick parade where hundreds of people are being pushed through..."

One of the solutions York discussed which would be very appropriate in the U.S. as well, is the use of health clinics staffed with a variety of health care professionals. The concept could be particularly effective in the rural areas and inner cities, but could also be applied to the suburbs. At one such clinic, cited as an example, most patients are treated by nurses and nurse practitioners. Social workers and other health professionals are also used as appropriate. In this way, only patients with more complex problems are sent to the doctors at the clinic. The result is that the doctors are able to spend more time with each patient they see. The patients can receive the time and personal attention they need since the responsibilities for patient care are dispersed among the various health professionals. The nurse practitioner is able to attend to many of the patient's basic care needs. Assistance is also provided by nursing personnel to help patients achieve healthier lifestyles and obtain good preventive care. Social workers and counselors help people deal more effectively with the pressures, stresses and decisions of daily life.

Not surprisingly, York noted that patients at the health center have been able to substantially reduce their use of mood altering drugs as well as the number of visits to the doctor. This type of community health center benefits everyone by keeping costs down and providing the patient with care matched to their specific needs. Unfortunately, development of these types of centers has not been encouraged on a widespread basis in Canada. Of course, this type of health care center is not appropriate for all situations, but there are many ways to incorporate these types of services into the health care system. President Clinton and Rep. Robert Michel strongly recommend expanding such community clinics in their plans.

While the Canadians are pleased with their system overall—polls show 85 to 90 percent approval rating—the system is undergoing some fundamental changes much like the U.S. because there is not enough money to pay for the system. At one time, Federal funding covered about *50 percent* of the health care costs in Canada. Now, due to the severe Canadian recession and spending levels which are rising nearly as fast as in the U.S., the Federal government is paying only 25 to 30 percent.

Furthermore, many of the provinces have actually been forced into deficit spending to finance health care. In some provinces, health care is consuming about one-third of the total spending available. There is some speculation that the current trend of dwindling Federal government outlay for contribution to the health care system will probably completely peter out by the end of the century and the provincial governments will be saddled with all of the health care expenses, according to C. Goar, in an article in *The Toronto Star*, February 23, 1991, "Budget Sure to Add to Provinces Burdens."

The problem is so serious that the largest province, Ontario, which has nearly 40 percent of the Canadian population, has cut back on many previously covered services. There have been tremendous cutbacks in hospital budgets and physicians' fees. Consequently, there are waiting lists for many procedures. It is common to wait nearly a year for a hip replacement surgery. Heart surgery is subject to an average wait of 23 weeks. The limitation of services is the primary fault Americans find with the Canadian system. It has become a common practice for patients to come to the U.S. in order to receive treatment in a more timely manner. The remarkable thing, however, is that Canadians seem to be coping with the situation quite well. Apparently, urgent care is generally provided within 24 hours in spite of the long wait for nonurgent care.

Those fascinated with the Canadian system should keep in mind that the U.S. federal government might do the same thing. We must guard against the U.S. government enacting a multitude of health care laws and guidelines for the states. As the budget continues to become a problem, the Federal government's financial support will necessarily dwindle causing the states to be saddled with an ever greater share of the nation's health care costs.

Health Care in Germany

"The old European tradition of carte blanche socialized medicine is tumbling to a new concept of cost control," says Timothy Harper in his article for *Medical Economics*, December 13, 1993, entitled, "Rationing, What We Can Learn From Europe." Budget restrictions are forcing European doctors to ration care as never before. They are using cost benefit analysis and fiscal implication of certain treatments to decide what treatments are most appropriate. This would open the eyes of people who look abroad and say that we should copy the systems of other industrialized countries.

The German system is experiencing difficult times. In the past, German hospitals, like many other systems worldwide, provided whatever care they considered appropriate and the government paid the bills. Today, because of severe financial restrictions, hospitals must carefully monitor their spending. Without openly declaring it, doctors are making rationing decisions about what treatment will be made available for each particular patient.

Harper gives a startling example of cost cutting measures being taken at the Michelsberg Klinik, a 190-bed pulmonary hospital in Bavaria. The director of the hospital and his staff now work an extra two to three hours every day. The extra hours are necessary to carefully analyze what is going to be spent on each patient. Decisions about what treatment—if any—will be given to each patient are based on the cost of treatment options and various factors such as the patient's age, prognosis and number of dependents, as well as personal habits, such as smoking, which may contribute to the patient's disease.

Because of new spending restrictions, German hospitals are on a tight budget. Budget increases are tied to the average national wage hike which is negotiated annually. In 1993, it was about three percent. Consequently, hospitals must limit what services can be provided which, according to Harper, "...puts doctors and administrators on a tight rope."

Failure to stay within the budget could mean government closure of the hospital. Failure to keep patients happy by providing the treatments they want may cause patients to seek care at other hospitals. If too many patients are dissatisfied, the loss of business would effectively close the hospital. To make matters worse, the staff is faced with extremely difficult decisions without at least having the benefit of formal guidelines or public consensus on the matter of rationing.

The long uncompensated hours and stressful decisions have caused many doctors to leave the hospitals where they were paid by salary to go into private practice. Physicians in private practice are paid through a fee-for-service system funded by payroll contributions to sickness funds. About 90 percent of Germans have coverage through a sickness fund. Costs to the sickness funds are controlled by regional caps. If too many services are rendered, the fee for each service decreases.

The employee payroll contribution to the sickness fund has been going up steadily in Germany. It has grown from an average of 12.2 percent of wages in 1991 to 12.6 percent in 1992. It was estimated to have reached 13.4 percent in 1993. Even with these increases, the government was forced to make up a $6 billion deficit in 1992. Health care costs in Germany are rising at a rate of about 10 percent per year, which is double the rate of inflation.

In addition to the spending restraints, it is interesting that the government has set a cap on the total cost of prescription drugs that can be ordered by an individual doctor or practitioner and has issued a mandatory age 68 retirement policy for most physicians. Patients also now pay a higher fee for a stay in the hospital.

Long waiting lists, as in other countries with limits on services, are becoming a reality in Germany. The government is adjusting the system's rules to try to keep costs down and minimize waits. Changes in the structure of sickness fund plans are allowing patients to choose their own fund. The government hopes this will encourage funds to utilize the hospitals with the lowest costs and offer coverage to its members at reduced rates. It has also been suggested to pay doctors a flat rate for a particular service and allow them to bargain with the hospitals for the lowest cost to utilize hospital facilities needed to provide the service.

In the end, all of the German government's solutions to combat rising health care costs come down to limiting costs while limiting service. Although people in Germany do not openly discuss rationing, it is a necessary reality in their health care system.

Health Care in the United Kingdom

Unlike Germany, the British have been openly discussing the problem of rationing. A recent British newspaper headline read, "Painful Dilemma of Who to Treat and not to Treat." The British Medical Association last year approved a resolution that termed rationing of health services an unfortunate fact of life. The resolution went even further to say that rationing should be done openly and doctors, "could not be held responsible for the consequences of political decisions about such rationing."

Health care spending in Britain currently stands at about 6.5 percent of the economy, up only one percentage point in 12 years. That appears to be the second lowest portion spent for health care in Western Europe, with Greece spending the lowest amount. While the British government boasts about these figures, most doctors consider this quite shameful and believe that spending seven to eight percent as other industrial countries do, would allow them to provide more services and trim the number of people in line for medical treatment from the current figure of nearly one million.

In England, rationing appears to occur in several ways. Waiting lists for services are one means of rationing. Another way rationing occurs is by denying some services or procedures to certain patients. The third is by denying certain treatments altogether. Health authorities have a waiting list, but the length varies from district to district and from hospital to hospital depending upon demand and what resources are available.

In order to "improve their system" there have been financial incentives provided to the hospitals over the past two years to become "trusts" that compete for business from district health authorities in terms of admissions from general practitioners. Similarly, the general practitioners have received incentives to become fund holders who receive annual capitation payments to cover their patient lists. They are then able to shop around for the best hospital bargains when they admit patients. While this has slightly reduced the waiting lists, it has created some problems for the hospitals. Instead of becoming all purpose local hospitals, they are specializing, expanding the services they can offer most efficiently and profitably and downgrading or dropping those services that are not cost effective.

This is compelling the family doctors not to consider what is best for their patients, but what would make their practice more financially successful. One doctor said his practice is building up patient participation groups to decide how the annual grant from National Health Service should be allocated. For example, they could discuss the virtue of using an expensive but effective treatment for acute migraine attack which would mean that the practice could afford one less hip operation or see 50 fewer outpatient appointments per year. It appears nobody has the answer to these problems and they are certainly not going to go away.

After carefully examining the health care systems of other countries, it is apparent that a wholesale adoption of any foreign plan is unlikely and would not work in America. We are more encouraged by the ability of Americans to solve their own health care problems without turning to other nations for solutions. In addition to the widely-publicized Clinton plan, there are already a diverse spectrum of proposals before Congress for health care reform. We will examine each briefly.

The Clinton Health Care Plan

Under President Clinton's plan for health care reform, all legal residents would be required to be insured, choosing from at least three plans providing standard benefits: a health maintenance organization, a fee-for-service plan or a combination plan. Clinton's plan will create large regional purchasing pools called health alliances. Everyone will be required to enroll in one of these alliances, which offer a variety of private health plans.

Clinton's plan guarantees universal coverage with a comprehensive package of benefits—although less generous than under the single-payer plan. He promises some coverage for mental health and substance abuse. Coverage for prescription drugs and limited long-term care will be added to Medicare benefits.

Employers will be required to pay 80 percent of insurance premiums for their workers, but no more than 7.9 percent of their payroll. Subsidies will be provided for small, low-wage employers. Individuals will pay up to 20 percent of their premiums. The fees of the poor will be subsidized.

Part of the financing of the Clinton plan includes new taxes of $105 billion on tobacco and large corporate employers who choose not to join regional purchasing alliances. If Clinton's plan is adopted, he promises reductions of $238 billion in anticipated growth of the Medicare and Medicaid programs from 1995 through 2000.

The Cooper Health Care Plan

Rep. Jim Cooper (D) of Tennessee, proposes managed competition. Like the Clinton Plan, everyone would be required to join a regional health alliance. These can include managed-care plans or traditional fee-for-service plans. The federal government would pay the insurance premiums for individuals below the poverty level and subsidize fees for individuals earning up to twice the poverty level.

Cooper's plan does not require employers to provide insurance but it allows the self-employed to deduct the full cost of standard insurance. Also, there would be no deductibles or co-payments allowed for preventive care. Policy cancellations and higher premium payments for pre-existing conditions, would be prohibited under the Cooper plan. Benefits would be set by a national health board.

Supporters say Cooper's plan will raise $16 billion by preventing employers from deducting the cost of insurance beyond the cost of basic plans, and another $6.5 billion by slowing Medicare increases.

The McDermott Single-Payer Plan

Supported by nearly one-third of the Democrats in the House, Rep. Jim McDermott (D) of Washington, proposes to replace the entire health insurance industry with a tax-financed system. The Federal government, acting as single-payer, would pay all medical bills, except extras such as private hospital rooms and cosmetic surgery. Individuals would never see a bill. The states would administer the system. This plan predicts massive savings in administrative costs since paperwork generated by the private health insurance industry is eliminated.

Substantial payroll taxes will be imposed on employers to fund the McDermott plan, but the theory is that employers will save some money by no longer having to supply their employees' health benefits.

The Chafee Plan

Senator John Chafee (R) of Rhode Island, with Senate support from both parties, would require all Americans to buy health insurance. Employers would be required to offer health plans to their employees but not necessarily pay any portion of the premiums. Individuals could also buy insurance through purchasing alliances. A national commission would determine a standard package of health benefits, including doctor and hospital services, prescription drugs, substance abuse and limited mental health coverage—offered at a reasonable cost. As the system produces savings, vouchers would be provided to the poor to subsidize their costs.

Chafee's plan will bar insurance companies from refusing coverage to people with pre-existing health problems. He argues that it would cut $213 billion in the growth of Medicare and Medicaid from 1995 through 2000. The plan will also limit tax deductibility of employer-paid insurance plans. The self-employed could deduct the full cost of standard health insurance.

The Michel Health Care Plan

Rep. Robert Michel (R) of Illinois offers a plan that would leave the current health insurance system largely unchanged. Employers would be required to offer their workers at least one insurance plan and a tax-free medical savings account or catastrophic policy. Deductibles for these catastrophic policies could be set at $1,800 or higher per person per year.

Michel proposes the expansion of community and migrant health care centers to increase access to care. Michel's plan promises to save $17 billion by reducing Medicare subsidies and altering Federal retirement rules.

The Gramm Health Care Plan

Sen. Phil Gramm (R) of Texas, encourages the use of insurance plans with very high deductibles that pay only "catastrophic" expenses. The supporters of the Gramm Plan are mostly conservative Republicans. Under this plan, employers would be required to offer workers at least three choices: the current health insurance plan, membership in an HMO or other provider, and a tax-free savings account to cover medical expenses that exceed $3,000 in a year. Employers must offer these insurance choices to their workers but are not required to pay for it. Families with less than 200 percent of poverty-level incomes, still not low enough to qualify for Medicaid, will get tax credits for their health care.

If put into action, Gramm says his plan will slow Medicaid growth by $113 billion and Medicare growth by $62 billion from 1994 to

1998. Lower business expenses would stimulate economic expansion resulting in an estimated $16 billion gain in revenues for the country.

Other Bipartisan Plans

Senator Don Nickles of Oklahoma and Rep. Cliff Stearns of Florida suggest that tax incentives be given to individuals to purchase insurance with a minimum standard benefit package. Their bill has about 40 co-sponsors.

Rep. Michael Bilirakis (D) of Florida and Rep. Roy Rowland (D) of Georgia, propose in their plan to end discrimination in the insurance system, while reforming the malpractice system. They want to automate the filing of insurance claims as well as expand the existence of community health centers. The representatives hope that their plan reduces health care costs without creating significant social change in the process. Their plan is supported by 17 Republicans and 17 Democrats.

Analyzing the Proposed Plans

After close scrutiny of all the currently proposed plans two major problems become clear. One group of plans would create an excessive new bureaucracy and require excessive new taxes, although they would definitely attempt to guarantee health care for all with a set of mandated benefits. The proposed regulations and methods to finance the health care under these plans cannot keep medical costs down for long and would lead to rationing and increased taxes, even though every effort is being made to prevent this eventuality.

The second group of proposals would be much less bureaucratic but leaves the situation relatively unchanged. They do not adequately address the problem of the uninsured but just hope that there will be sufficient savings and when these savings accrue, the uninsured would be taken care of. A subset of the second group of plans touches on the concept of "Medisave" which appears very appealing. We will deal with this concept in greater detail later in this chapter.

A recent poll taken by the *Los Angeles Times* showed that about 70 percent of people state, categorically, that they would understand if

Congress is unable to pass a health care reform bill this year. People are more concerned that when Congress does pass a health care reform bill, they do it right and not just come up with something to beat the clock. In this analysis, we will touch on the major drawbacks of some of the leading plans and then select some of the best aspects of the various plans, merge them together and hopefully come up with a solution which is much simpler, easier to administer, and more effective in achieving the goals set out by the President—namely, controlling costs and providing health care for every American who wants it.

The major problem the lawmakers are facing right now is how to find the money to meet the health care needs of all Americans, especially the 37 million who are uninsured, without busting the precarious budget. Various tax proposals have been suggested, unfortunately additional taxes is really the wrong remedy for the health care crisis. The American health care crisis is due primarily to uncontrollable spending, not too little money being spent. Therefore, any reform that adds more money to an already bloated expenditure is not a step in the right direction. Unfortunately, one influential Congressional committee chairman has so much as said that a substantial tax increase would be needed to provide insurance for the uninsured.

One tax proposal is to exempt employers with less than 10 workers and charge companies with 10 to 20 workers a one to two percent payroll tax. Another idea being seriously considered is to tax employee health benefits, at least partially. One expert claims that it would raise revenue and also control costs. Some who are vehemently opposed to employer mandates state that they are neutral on taxing employee health benefits. However, taxes on employee's health benefits would have just the same adverse effect on employees as companies would suffer under employer mandates. Employee benefit taxes are wrong for the following reasons. The major reason is that they are not needed and create undue financial burdens on the middle class, whose income has either fallen or been stagnant the last several years. Most current insurance plans have a $100 to $250 deductible. Most expenses, after some co-payment, are fully covered. Therefore, after the deductible and co-payment has been met, the patient may feel entitled to use the coverage even more. Taxing part of the insurance premium would only give the consumer more incentive to use the coverage as much as possible, because if they do not use it before the year is over, the contribution is lost forever. Unfortunately, once part of the health care premium, say 25 percent, is taxed without public outcry, the next year or the year after, 20 percent more will be taxed since the revenue generated would never be sufficient to cover all the mandated benefits. Before long 50 to 75 percent or even 100 percent of the health benefits would be in danger of being taxed. Consider, for example, a Chrysler employee whose health care contribution is currently about $6000. We propose that instead of taking $1000 in taxes, we reward the individual consumer with $1000 to $1500 in a savings plan or some form of account for the employee if they use their health care benefits prudently. They should have part of the benefits of their savings to encourage them to become educated and economical consumers.

Another problem with several of the Congressional proposals is that the employer must offer the employee some form of insurance but the employer does not have to pay for it. This simply will not help the uninsured employee. If they are offered insurance and they cannot afford it, what good does it do them? These proposals are just a variation of the current COBRA plan which mandates the employer to offer an ex-employee up to 18 months of insurance which the employee can purchase on his own. It is a fact that the majority, over 50 percent, of the uninsured and unemployed are in this group. The suggestion that the employer should offer coverage but not pay for it would probably encourage more employers not to cover their employees. They would feel they have fulfilled their legal obligation by simply making insurance available without paying for it. Therefore, this might actually increase the number of uninsured, at least temporarily. I am not advocating employer mandate, I am simply pointing out the hollowness of the concept of the employer providing but not paying for insurance.

Third, many of the proposals for saving money rely on a theoretical possibility of reducing only the *growth* of health care outlay. Many of the Congressional proposals would use this phantom savings, which most likely will never materialize, to cover the uninsured at some future time when the savings is realized. Congressional leaders have toiled long and hard over the decade without much success using the same tools to control Medicare costs. It is, therefore, unlikely that some miracle would occur that would release a huge new savings.

These three problems are part of the reason why the lawmakers are still having such a hard time drafting any meaningful health care legislation. There is really no way to come up with a health care solution with the current proposals in Congress without raising taxes substantially. Mr. Dan Rostenkowski, former Chairman of The House Ways and Means Committee, was quoted on May 11, 1994, as saying, "If someone can show me how we can fill what I estimate to be a $40 billion hole in the year 2000, I will be glad to listen." This is why Mr. Rostenkowski continued to defend his call for a broad-based tax to help pay for universal health care coverage. Mr. Clinton is wise to say that this type of tax would not be sound or fair.

The Medisave Alternative

The Medisave concept has been touted by several groups as a means of reducing unnecessary use of services. However, it has not been properly brought to the forefront of health care reform discussions. This plan gives the patient financial incentive to cut health care cost—some claim by as much as 25 percent—without reducing quality. The current system works this way: the employer pays a premium of $4000 to $4500 per year to the insurance company for a plan with a $100 to $200 deductible and a small co-payment. With Medisave, individuals get a tax incentive to buy insurance with a high deductible of $3000 but pay a premium as low as $1500. The employer puts the other $3000 that would have been spent in a tax-free medical savings account. This $3000 could be used to pay for deductible covered medical expenses.

It has been proven that most patients will have lots of money left over at the end of the year and can save this money for health coverage if they lose their jobs or their health benefits run out. Medisave would also be an effective way of reducing unnecessary procedures because it puts the patient in charge of policing his/her own care.

There are those who argue that the patient will delay medical treatment to save money. However, this concept has already been put in effect by a small number of companies and delaying or avoiding care has not been shown to be a problem.

A closer look at these results make this option extremely appealing and it will save a considerable amount of money, if available nationwide. It is estimated that spending under the current trend will be $540 billion in 1995 and will rise to $775 billion in 1997 for people *under* 65 years old. However, with the Medical Savings Plan the outlay will be $430 billion in 1995 and $490 billion in 1997. This represents a substantial savings.

Two articles from *Investor's Business Daily*, May 20, 1993 and March 18, 1994, entitled, "Letting Employees Rein In the Costs" by Chris Warden and "Employees as Health

Premium Costs
(Under Age 65)

Costs are in Billions of Dollars

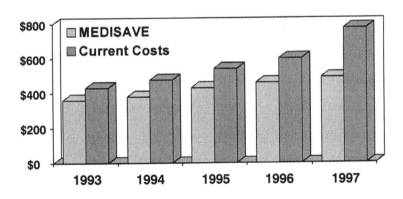

Data: Council for Affordable Insurance (*Investor's Business Daily*, 3/18/94).

Reformers," by John Merline discuss some versions of the Medisave plan.

The articles dismiss the widely-held belief that medical costs are not like other markets and competition does not bring down prices. J. Kennerly Davis, Vice President of Dominion Resources Utility Holding Company in Richmond, however, asserts that a market is a market and the outcome of transactions in a market would be efficient and equitable as long as you get the right incentives. He added that people are rational and are perfectly capable of making decisions regarding their own affairs and finances. Under this premise, Dominion set up an incentive plan to encourage employees to be prudent and careful consumers of health care dollars.

Under the plan called "Share the Savings," the employees choose a plan with either low deductible and higher monthly premiums or a high deductible with lower monthly premiums. Those who choose a high deductible and do not use the full deductible, receive bonus dollars at the end of the year. In addition, they build a medical savings account arising from the low monthly premiums. About 75 percent of the employees are voluntarily enrolled in the low premium, high deductible plans. Premiums are as low as $1500 per year with a deductible of $1500 per individual or $3000 per family. The employees are given sufficient money to cover their deductible expenses. If they do not spend the entire amount available for deductible, they get the remainder as a bonus. Last year, most high deductible plan enrollees received a bonus of about $800. In addition, the savings from the premiums are put into a health care savings account for the employees and are immediately vested.

Because of these innovative techniques which let the consumer control health care spending, health care costs for Dominion have gone up by less than one percent since 1989. Compare this with the 10 to 13 percent annual increase in spending nationwide. Dominion also has a wellness program including $50 a month to encourage participants to take care of their medical problems promptly and participate in preventive programs.

Golden Rule Insurance Company has a similar plan in effect. Whatever money employees with a high deductible don't spend, they keep. Last year employees received $470,000 in bonuses with 80 percent of employees voluntarily participating in the plan.

Forbes Publishing Co. also has an incentive plan in place with impressive savings. The company paid up to $1000 bonus to over 500 employees who filed claims sparingly. Claims have dropped by 30 percent in dollar amount and the number of claims filed has declined by 20 percent.

In 1993, the Council of Affordable Health Insurance *switched* from a managed care plan with a $250 deductible to a fee-for-service plan with a $1000 deductible and savings available for workers if they do not spend it. Their premium went up only 4.6 percent in 1994. One satisfied employee noted that she had enough money left over for preventive care and still received a bonus of $760 in December 1993.

Dr. Peter Somani, Director of the Ohio Department of Health, estimates that by switching to a Medisave-type plan, the State could save at least $29 million annually with only one-half of State's employees enrolled in the plan. He feels this is a conservative estimate since it does not include savings that will accrue form resulting changes in the health care consumption habits of employees.

Patient Friendly Medisave

This is different from a simple catastrophic policy. This Medisave plan actually will provide sufficient money to cover practically all deductible and co-payments but at the same time ensure that the money is spent prudently. The legitimate concern about mere catastrophic policies is that people who cannot afford the high deductible will simply not seek help. In fact, Medisave will be superior to the traditional policies which still leave families with a $250 to $600 deductible that they must pay out of their pocket in order to access their current coverage.

Incorporating these types of concepts into our health care system will provide patients with the incentive needed to help control their own costs. It will be beneficial to businesses, both large and small, in that it will stabilize the ballooning cost of providing health care benefits. In the remaining chapters, we will address the insurance industry's role in initiating the momemtum for reform, review the key elements of the agenda for reform and examine how those components can work together to achieve the desired goals.

CHAPTER 6

Cost Control Measures Begin To Pay Off

Before we discuss specific solutions to the health care crisis, it is worthwhile to examine some of the achievements that have already occurred in health care cost reduction. Substantial cost reduction is a prerequisite for greater health care access. This is an important chapter because it will show that there is indeed reason to believe that health care costs can be controlled. In many areas the cost has really tumbled. Industry and individuals must start demanding a share of these profits from the insurance companies. We should not be satisfied with a health care inflation rate of eight percent in 1994 when the general rate of inflation was only three percent.

An article in the December 8, 1994 issue of *Investor's Business Daily* reports that HMO enrollment accelerated during the first nine months of 1994 with more than five million new enrollees bringing the total to 50 million people. The Group Health Association of America surveyed about 70 HMO's and predicted a 1.2 percent reduction in premium costs for 1995. This is still not enough cost reduction considering all the current and potential tools that are available through free enterprise to reduce costs.

The Strength of Free Market Forces

The effectiveness of free enterprise forces is illustrated in a very informative article in *Medical Economics* (July 11, 1994) in which

Anita Slomski discussed "How Business is Flattening Health Costs". A self-insured corporation refused to pay for a failed kidney transplant until the hospital discounted the bill $500,000. The corporation agreed to pay $800,000 for the failed transplant. The same company reduced their health care costs by 2.8 percent in 1993, saving $2.2 million. They expected to reduce it another five percent in 1994.

Helen Darling, corporate benefits manager of Xerox, states that the medical industry is used to 18 percent inflation, hence they think that eight percent is a big improvement. Xerox is eliminating 10,000 jobs worldwide and provided no merit raises in 1994. She complained that medical inflation is still 1.5–2.5 times the Consumer Price Index (CPI). Therefore, an eight percent increase, or any increase, is unacceptable.

A PepsiCo executive was elated that he had reduced health care inflation to five percent, but the company chairman rightfully demanded that the new target should be zero increase without cutting benefits or quality.

Slomski also pointed out that not only are large firms demanding and getting cost reduction throughout the country, but many small businesses are forming coalitions and exclusive networks of providers. In Houston, a group of eight companies has convinced 40 hospitals to accept a uniform fee schedule with heavy discounts of 35 - 40 percent. One hospital that failed to sign up initially was experiencing a loss of physician loyalty and subsequently, a large number of empty beds. They decided to join the plan. This was the first time that this particular hospital signed a major managed care contract.

This arrangement has virtually wiped out any cost shifting to offset the discount hospitals give to managed care plans. But this coalition went even further. In order to change doctors' habits, they expect to pay the identical fee for a C-section delivery as a vaginal birth to reduce Houston's 33 percent C-section rate to the national average of 24 percent.

The business group expects to put all these hospitals on quasi-probation for two years and closely monitor performance. Those that don't measure up to quality standards set by a committee of local doctors will be eliminated. The same probation period applies to physicians. After a trial period, doctors whose quality is not up to par will be dropped. Ralph Smith, the chairman of the coalition, said that they hold physicians accountable just like anyone else in business.

This project has worked very well so far because the coalition has repeatedly sought and obtained physician input on the arrangement on all levels. A physician chairman of the county medical society socio-economic committee remarked that the coalition realizes that they don't gain anything by driving fees so low as to bankrupt doctors. Also, by eliminating the middle man, i.e. the insurer, the coalition of businesses has been able to give a little more to the providers.

Employers are also taking a serious look at HMO's and demanding high quality at affordable rates. They scrutinize the plan's financial stability, membership turnover and preventive treatment program. In addition, they evaluate the qualifications of doctors and the number of specialists in the HMO and conduct thorough patient satisfaction surveys. Most companies take all these factors into account when choosing an HMO.

The Downside of Insensitive Cost Reduction Techniques

While industry has been instrumental in demanding cost reduction and increasing quality, the insurance industry still controls the bulk of care provided in the U.S. The insurance companies are now in the best position to control health care costs. They are demanding effective cost control measures from providers and getting them. The real question is will they pass on the savings to employers and consumers or spend the profits to acquire competitors at exorbitant prices and make strategic alliances.

The insurance companies are now in the same position doctors and hospitals were in seven to fifteen years ago when they had virtual autonomy. At that time, providers could charge whatever they felt was appropriate and insurance companies paid it. Then doctors and other providers had too much control and some definitely abused the system. Bruce Karrh, occupational medicine specialist and vice-president of DuPont's integrated health care program, observed that

"Physicians had the opportunity to control the way care is delivered, but they didn't take it. So other parties took on the role." The tables have now turned. In some cases, however, we have gone to the opposite extreme. Many insurance companies now determine a payment schedule on a "take it or leave it" basis which is, at times, below the cost of providing the care.

In the current environment, insurance companies' control of doctors and hospitals ranges from a reasonable working relationship to a ludicrous arrangement which may be outright detrimental to the welfare of patients. The best companies thoroughly research the track record of their selected providers, allowing them to perform their duties without constant interference unless there is a deviation from acceptable patterns of care. Other companies want to control every step of patient care with little regard for the welfare of the patient. The following real-life cases illustrate some of the ways insurance companies hinder patients from receiving the appropriate care.

A medical director for an insurance company demanded chemotherapy be stopped after six months on a 32-year-old woman with breast cancer. The oncologist explained that this was not an ordinary case. The patient had a poorer prognosis because she is young and had an aggressive tumor that was estrogen receptor negative. The doctor felt strongly that longer treatment was warranted. The patient was reluctant to continue chemotherapy unless the medical director approved coverage for it for financial reasons. The oncologist told the medical director that he could stop the chemotherapy but would have to write a note to the patient stating that further chemotherapy was recommended but the medical director refused to approve it. Only at this point did the director reluctantly approved further treatment but still threatened the oncologist with expulsion from the program if he did not conform to "cook-book" cancer treatment. Is this the way we want decisions about our health care to be made?

A 34-year-old male developed a serious hematological condition in which his body was literally chewing up his own red blood cells and platelets. His hematocrit fell to 15 percent from a normal level of 45 percent and his platelet count dropped to 5,000 from a normal of about 400,000. After numerous telephone consultations with other specialists from a major teaching hospital, for which there is no charge to the patient, the patient became stabilized and was discharged. However, in order to understand exactly what was going on and prevent future relapse, it was felt that the patient should be sent for a formal consultation with another specialist at a teaching hospital to find out the exact nature of his condition. Although the specialist worked at a network institution, the assistant to the medical director requested that detailed records be submitted for his evaluation before they could approve the consultation. Despite the seriousness of the patient's condition, the assistant to the medical director said that it might take about a week to make a decision. After two days of frustration, wasting another two hours on the phone on the third day and sending numerous faxes of the patient's records, they approved a limited consultation, i.e. the patient could receive advice only, no testing would be allowed. The case was highly complex and required input from a team of doctors who carefully researched the case and prepared a six-page report with a presumptive diagnosis which concurred with the ongoing treatment. The patient has remained free of further problems for the time being.

The same insurance company frustrated another patient who is a supervisor at a major corporation in the computer and defense industry. The patient was diagnosed with breast cancer on a Friday. However, because of a very bad snowstorm, no one of authority was available in the insurance office that day to approve the surgery on the weekend, so the patient and doctor had to wait until the next week to obtain permission for her surgery, although there was no doubt about the necessity of the operation. In surgery, the patient chose immediate reconstruction which was performed by a competent plastic surgeon on the staff. The patient was not aware that this plastic surgeon was not on her insurance list. She had to pay for the reconstruction out of her own pocket since the insurance company refused to pay for it. The insurance company should have paid for the reconstruction up to the level they normally approve and the patient should be responsible for anything above the customary rate.

Due to their dissatisfaction with the manner in which the insurance company handled their access to care, these two patients left this insurance company as soon as their employer offered a new enrollment period that allowed them to switch to another plan. This supervisor is certain her company will drop this particular insurance company at the earliest opportunity because of numerous other complaints by other employees.

This insurance company happens to be a rapidly growing company due to heavy marketing and slightly lower initial costs to employers. They claim to have a patient satisfaction rate of over 90 percent. However, I seriously doubt the validity of the survey and their ability to maintain their volume of enrollment without providing genuine satisfaction to their patients.

Another situation that was frustrating for both the patient and doctor involved a young man with recurrent tonsil and ear infections. The patient had received frequent antibiotic therapy for a long time. He began to have hearing loss and difficulty with learning. The ENT (Ear, Nose and Throat) specialist felt they had tried antibiotics long enough and the patient should have a tonsillectomy. The insurance representative, however, decided that the patient should be on antibiotics for at least three months to be considered eligible for surgery. After much frustration, the mother gave the go ahead for surgery. She felt her son needed to have the surgery and she would rather pay for it and fight the insurance company later. There should be a better method of determining medical necessity for procedures which have been known to have a high volume, such as tonsillectomy. There is an obvious need to establish effective means of reducing unnecessary procedures without causing undue problems for patients. There is, however, no justification to use these criteria as a means of denying coverage arbitrarily.

Another insurance company was requesting frequent phone updates on a patient because she was on a case management plan. The physician's office literally had to spell every third word to the secretary who then relayed the information to those making the decisions about approving care. One day she asked for the spelling of the word "CBC" (Complete Blood Count). This is like a law office asking help to spell "UCC" (Uniform Commercial Code). Far too often, unqualified insurance personnel cause unnecessary delays and frustrations wasting the time of valuable personnel in the doctor's office or hospital, while allowing the insurance company to increase their profit margins through the use of low-cost clerical workers.

The insurance companies now have a virtual monopoly over deciding when patients can be admitted to the hospital and how long they can stay. Even if they approve the stay in advance, they can later deny it or only pay for a portion of the hospital stay. If all or part of the hospital care is denied, the only recourse is to make an appeal to the same company to reverse their decision. Invariably, however, they stick to the original decision. This often arbitrary refusal to pay for in-hospital services after the fact has cost hospitals millions and produces huge savings for some insurance companies. This situation could be compared to the police issuing a policy, making arrests based on the policy, prosecuting the case, rendering judgement and hearing the appeal. This is a preposterous scenario but, unfortunately, it occurs far too often in the insurance industry The top health insurance executives are probably not even aware of these problems.

Often much of the cost containment enforcement is contracted out to emerging consulting companies which spring up all over, many of which really do not understand the actual causes of escalating health care costs. While they fail to pay for legitimate services which will, in the long run, be more beneficial to the patient and save other costly expenditures, they are paying billions without question for services which are of far more limited value. This short-sightedness is a fundamental issue of quality versus quantity that must be addressed by all insurance carriers. Otherwise the payment process will continue to frustrate and penalize superior doctors and hospitals and reward those whose strategy for survival is to increase the volume of their work whether necessary or not.

In an article in *Oncology Times* (Dec. 1994, p. 8), Ruth SoRelle, MPH wrote that the future is uncertain for MD Anderson Hospital. While the hospital had nearly a four percent increase in patient load in 1993, revenues were down ten percent. They had to cut $30 million from the $586 million budget to reduce expenses. They plan to directly lay off 180 people and eliminate more by attrition, thereby reducing the work force by five percent. More lay offs are planned for the future. Charles LeMaistre, President of the institution, states labor costs account for one-half of the hospital's total costs. He finds it difficult to lay off people who are doing their job well, however, he feels that if the hospital does not increase revenues aggressively and cut costs, they will be out of business in two years.

Another problem facing individuals as well as institutions is providing an ever increasing number of uncompensated services. The state of Texas provides MD Anderson Cancer Center $108 million annually and requires it to provide cancer care to Texans even if they cannot pay. This $108 million has not increased for nearly ten years. Yet the hospital provided $200 million of uncompensated care to the indigent in 1993. The famed Memorial Sloane Kettering Cancer Center is in a similar situation. They are closing one floor to eliminate 45 beds and reduce staff size by 300 with 70 direct lay offs and the remainder through attrition.

In the past, this short fall in coverage for uncompensated care would easily have been made up by charging higher amounts to private insurance companies. The increasing influence of managed care has now eliminated most of this inequitable cost shifting. However, we have not solved the problem of paying for the cost of care provided to uninsured patients. Managed care has merely shifted the burden to another group in the health care equation. Large hospitals are not the only ones feeling the pinch. Most hospitals are either being sold or have joined forces with others to stay afloat because of the tight squeeze.

Achieving Further Cost Reduction Without Reduction in Quality

A large insurance company demanded a 15 percent discount from a very successful and efficient health care provider. The profit margin was greatly reduced but the provider was still able to cover costs successfully by being more cost effective. The provider started printing the discount they gave the insurance company on the patient bills in order to arrive at the amount of the patient's portion of the bill. However, the insurance company threatened to cancel their contract if the provider did not stop revealing the substantial discount being given to the insurance company. The American public has not yet realized that the insurance industry is reaping substantial reward from the aggressive efforts being made by industry and the public to control health care costs. Patient welfare may be seriously compromised at times, while doctors and hospitals are sometimes paid less than the cost of the service they provide.

Attorney Noah Rosenberg of Beverly Hills complained that insurance companies are spreading financial risks but not profit to doctors. He noted that doctors are getting "shafted" by the insurance industry in an article by Bruce Jances in *Internal Medicine News and Cardiology* (December 1, 1994). The insurance industry has asked doctors to assume greater financial risk in providing health care and at the same time provide enormous savings to the insurance industry. He suggested that doctors should properly organize to rectify the situation since no one else can practice medicine. Doctors in many states are organizing physician-owned HMOs in order to maintain a better balance. Even though the average length of stay in hospitals has significantly decreased over the last few years, doctors, hospitals and industry have not seen a cent of savings passed on to them. Insurance companies are also getting a tremendous break on outpatient services, but again, premium costs do not reflect these savings.

Direct deal-making by industry and insurance companies with doctors, hospitals and pharmaceutical companies is leading to the creation of effective, informal alliances. Through free market principles, even a small step, such as the one taken by Lubrizol, has led to huge savings.

According to an article by Geoffrey Leavenworth in *Business & Health*, August 1994, Lubrizol had a 12 percent annual health care cost increase for five years until 1992. In 1993, they had an increase of only 0.8 percent, and a savings of about $1.2 million. Lubrizol achieved this remarkable savings by contracting directly with physicians and hospitals in Cleveland and Houston. While many companies are scrambling to cut deals to save money, Lubrizol is interested in both quality of care as well as the reduction of cost. This arrangement is attractive for industry and providers because industry benefits from cost reduction and preferred providers have the opportunity for an attractive steady patient load.

Direct contracting for laboratory and x-ray services is becoming commonplace. For example, Lubrizol's lab and x-ray costs exploded from $700,000 to $1.2 million in 1992. By lab contracting, they have significantly reduced the cost. However, when improperly arranged, these contracts have become very burdensome to both providers and the insured.

Savings Produced at the Patient's Expense

A very large nationwide corporation has contracted with a single preferred laboratory for all services. Patients must go to one of a small number of testing sites to have blood samples taken. These centers are inconvenient for the patient since they must usually travel considerable distance to get to the nearest location. In addition, the staff in some of these centers are not highly skilled and are frequently unable to obtain the necessary blood samples causing the patient unnecessary trauma. The lab contract has been modified to allow some medical specialties to perform the blood testing at their own location when test results are needed more urgently. However, the provider is penalized for needing the lab results more promptly since payment under the lab contract for a profile of 25 blood tests is about $3.00 while other managed care plans pay about $15.00 for the same set of tests.

One major insurance company has demanded that all patients go to only approved x-ray facilities. However, they have only contracted with small, independent facilities offering limited services. These facilities are very willing to accept an exceedingly low payment in return for expecting a greatly increased volume of business. As a result, patients must go to several different facilities all over town in order to obtain a chest x-ray at one place, and ultrasound or CAT scanning procedures at other locations. This type of edict is made without any thought of the consequences for patient care. To have the patient go to different parts of town for different x-rays makes it impossible to compare current x-ray films with CAT scans and, worse yet, it becomes impossible to compare current films with old films which is especially critical in the management of cancer patients.

Such ill-conceived plans cut dollars off the bottom line for the insurance company, but increase costs and time expenditure for patients and physicians and have an extremely negative impact on the quality of care. When quality is compromised to achieve maximum dollars of savings, the net result is not a savings for the health care system overall but rather a shifting of the burden.

We have taken the time to give you these examples not to diminish the excellent quality service most health insurance companies are providing but to alert industry and the public about some of the pitfalls and to demand solutions before they get out of control. Typically, these companies offer numerous health plans. It is the responsibility of the insurance company executives to carefully evaluate the plans they offer and not make choices based solely on cost.

Controversies in Insurance Reform

Because of the complexity and myriad of insurance products, insurance reform will not be an easy task. There are many controversial areas where full guaranteed access to a particular medical procedure will be detrimental to the insurance industry. Bone marrow transplant treatment for breast cancer, for example, is being used even at present without strict selection criteria for people who will benefit. Mandatory coverage for bone marrow transplant as treatment for breast cancer will simply lead to explosive usage which may not necessarily increase cure rates.

Another controversial area which must be dealt with equitably involves pre-existing conditions. The following example illustrates the dilemma faced by millions. A 50-year-old woman had cancer of the breast and received chemotherapy. The cancer was in remission and she had moved to live with her mother who had Alzheimer's Disease, as well as breast cancer which was in remission. A year later, the daughter developed a recurrence of her cancer on the chest wall and in the bone. She began receiving more chemotherapy which included one of the most useful, but very expensive, chemotherapy medications called Novantrone. One vial costs over $600. Unfortunately, she lost her job. She did find a new job, but the new insurance company did not cover her pre-existing condition of breast cancer. There was a one year exclusion provision for pre-existing conditions. Her solution was to stop chemotherapy until her insurance would cover her breast cancer condition. Obviously, this was not a viable option.

The pharmaceutical company assumed responsibility for the necessary medication and provided the doctor with enough Novantrone at no charge for this patient to complete her treatment. When pre-existing conditions are excluded from coverage, the patient is usually still able to get treatment by various assistance programs or discounts. However, our suggestion to modify the COBRA program to extend coverage when one loses their job for a period of time will go a long way towards a solution for coverage in such situations. (See Chapter 7 for a discussion of this concept.)

While examples such as the above should be covered, it would not be fair to force insurance companies to fully cover those who refuse to pay for insurance coverage under a regular plan when they suddenly get sick. We don't allow people to go without auto insurance until they sustain a crash and then allow them to buy insurance to include their previous collision. Even though the same principles should apply regarding health insurance, it is not that simple. When someone is bleeding or gasping for air, you don't ask about insurance; you simply take care of the patient first.

Another problem is arbitrary termination of insurance coverage. A very hard-working, extremely pleasant patient had an aggressive tumor which was no longer responsive to surgery, radiation or chemotherapy. The man could hardly breathe because of the extensive tumor in his chest but he continued to work until two months before his death because he adamantly claimed that his policy stipulated that he would lose his insurance coverage the day he quit work. He did not want to leave his wife with huge medical bills. His oncologist offered to write or talk to his boss who runs a very successful medium-sized company, but the patient felt it would do no good. When he finally could not make it to work, he approached his boss who was immediately supportive and took care of the medical bills including hospice care. This is where Medisave could have made a difference. Regulations must protect the insured from arbitrary suspension of benefits due to circumstances beyond their control.

The type and scope of coverage in insurance policies is another problem area. Coverage ranges from skeletal or bare bones coverage, which hardly protects the individual and requires a huge amount of out of pocket payment, to the other extreme of excessive coverage— so-called "gold-plated" plans. Lawmakers must guard against mandating such gold-plated coverage which becomes too expensive, especially for those between the ages of 18–26 who will simply fail to buy insurance altogether because they can't afford it. This is another glaring example of unfounded state and federal mandates for individuals.

Emerging Dominance of Managed Care

In 1991, two-thirds of all office-based doctors participated in managed care. By 1993, the number had risen to three-fourths. In 1991, HMO and PPO groups combined accounted for 22 percent of the typical doctor's income. By 1993, 38 percent of the doctor's income came from HMO or PPO plans but the doctor's income from *all* sources during that same period had increased by less than 2 percent. These figures indicate the large shift from traditional insurance plans to managed care.

As a greater percentage of care shifts from traditional plans to managed care, the insurance company has the power to choose and reject providers at will. They can arbitrarily terminate the physician's ability to provide care for their patients at any time without explanation. To guard against such situations, some medical societies are urging Congress to pass a law that any interested qualified provider should be included in each plan and that reasons to terminate a provider must be explicit. Many insurance companies argue that they only reject five to ten percent of the providers whom they strictly investigate for selection during their credentialling process. A provision to allow any willing provider to participate in a network will, in effect, negate the advantage of the physician giving the insurance company a deep discount in exchange for an assumed increase in volume of patients.

Caution about Capitation

There should also be protection for the individual, as well as industry, when an insurance company's or a provider's incompetent, reckless actions lead to bankruptcy causing undue burden on the insured who are left without coverage. One of the unpredictable tools currently being used to control health care costs is capitation. This is really an area where "fools rush in where angels fear to tread". Many providers have been badly burnt, leaving patients without doctors or insurance coverage.

Capitation works this way: the providers are paid some monthly stipend to take care of stipulated health care needs of a number of clients. If the client population does not consume a lot of health care dollars, the provider makes money. However, if the provider has too many sick patients or is not efficient, he loses money. With a large group of providers, the risks of capitated payment are spread around. However, with a small group of providers, one or a few very sick patients can literally wipe out any possibility of profit in a capitated arrangement. This has led to several bankrupt groups, leaving their patients stranded.

Unfortunately, many small groups are springing up to sign up for capitated arrangements that are doomed to fail from the start for several reasons. First, the group is too small to absorb even a few catastrophic illnesses. Second, the providers are not business people and are totally inexperienced in managing such an arrangement. Third, many groups don't have the sophisticated computer and support systems necessary to track what is going on financially with their company. They take current premiums to pay past claims and as long as the provider group is growing with more new contracts, it will do fine. But once it stops growing, the cushion dries up. Unless they are on sound financial footing, they will run into problems. There is such fierce competition among providers to land contracts with insurance companies that they don't analyze the financial risks well enough to see whether they have a viable contract. Lauren M. Walker, Senior Associate Editor of *Medical Economics* described one large capitated group in California that went bankrupt due mainly to inexperience and lack of foresight (December 12, 1994). He quoted the associate director of the failed provider group saying, "We did not understand capitation well enough." What an understatement!

One of the other major factors in causing the failure of capitated groups is that doctors are still practicing as though they are in a fee-for-service arrangement. Also, the insurance company unloaded most of the risks on the providers while taking a disproportionate percentage of the premium income. The arrangements most likely to succeed are those orchestrated directly between industry and providers where quality comes first or at least quality and cost are put on equal footing. Industry and the public should be very careful about paying large premiums to insurance companies to dabble in capitated arrangements with little guarantee for success.

Health Care Inflation Down — But Not Enough

The health care inflation rate in 1993 was 7.8 percent and 1994's estimated rate was 8.0 percent. Although reduced from earlier years, this level is still two to three times higher than the general rate of inflation and is intolerable in times when maximum effort is being made by a large segment of the population to reduce costs. If eight percent health care inflation is the best we can do with maximum effort, then we are really in deep trouble. If the other reform measures presented in this book are instituted, there is no reason we cannot see a 10–20 percent reduction in overall costs in a very short time. Industry and the public at large should, at that point, demand a share of that savings.

The good new is costs are coming down by and large without reducing quality. The better news is quality has become the number one concern. At the same time, a more substantial cost reduction for industry is still achievable. Ralph R. Smith, Jr., director of employee benefits for Mitchell Energy & Development in Houston, sums it up in the July 11, 1994 issue of *Medical Economics* stating, "Now we're saying to providers give us an appropriate amount of medicine in the appropriate setting with good outcome, and we'll pay a reasonable price for it. I'm willing to pay more for quality—though I believe it costs less in the long run."

Insurance Premium Reduction of 10–20 Percent Achievable

A most informative article by George Anders in *The Wall Street Journal*, 12/21/94 vindicated the two salient points of this book:
1. There is already too much money in the health care system and no more money needs to be added to provide insurance coverage for everyone.
2. Medical insurance premiums are too high and can be reduced at least 25 percent without jeopardizing the quality of care.

Even with substantial premium reductions, a medical savings plan can work to help consumers and employers without crippling the insurance industry. The current pricing of health insurance effectively charges the customer the equivalent of whole life insurance premiums and gives them the equivalent of term life benefits.

HMO's in Unique Financial Position

The *Wall Street Journal* article is appropriately entitled "Money Machines: HMO's Pile Up Billions in Cash, Try to Decide What to Do With It." The liquid assets of many HMO's increased 15 percent last year and nine of the largest HMO's have a combined total of over $9.5 billion excess cash. Each of the four largest HMO's have over $1 billion stuck away and many mid-sized HMO's have over one-half billion dollars free cash. Because of rapid membership growth and reduced medical costs, many HMO's are accumulating money faster than they know how to spend it. Anders quoted one officer for an HMO with headquarters in Pueblo, Colorado as saying "Our problem is what to do with the money that comes in, *not* whether we have enough cash." This HMO has one-half billion dollars cash and is *increasing its cash position by $500,000 daily!* The astronomical influx of cash is making it exceedingly difficult for the treasurer of this HMO to find places to invest the money, e.g. treasury bills, certificates of deposit and other short-term investments. The HMO with the largest cash position has $2.6 billion. An executive with this company boasts that "people always want to know what we are going to do with [the cash]. We're in no hurry. And until we know, people will just have to guess."

A California HMO in Woodland Hills with a mere 0.7 million members reportedly has $1.9 billion in "cash." "Cash" is defined as bank deposits or any marketable security with a maturity of one year or less. With a recent stock price of $28 per share, cash accounted for $19 of the value per share. Similarly, a Milwaukee HMO with a stock price of $34 has $32 per share of its value in cash. Ms. Vignola notes that with the increase in interest rates, most HMO's might keep the reserves invested in conservative short-term vehicles. Consequently, many will report substantial investment income in 1995, perhaps as high as 10 percent of operating earnings.

Why are HMO's suddenly so wealthy? First of all, HMO's direct their patients to selected doctors and providers considered most cost-efficient. Any savvy business man can set up a successful HMO. Since premiums are used to pay for expenses, after a small amount of initial start-up capital, very little additional capital is necessary to grow. No factories or heavy equipment is needed. HMO's are now in a position to dictate the terms of "employment" to the providers. The HMO's are able to "cherry pick" all the healthy working people who hardly get sick. Remember, the healthiest 50 percent of Americans consume only three percent of the health care dollars. This is why it is possible for a small HMO in an affluent area in California with only 0.7 million subscribers to amass $1.9 billion in cash reserves in a few years.

Margo Vignola, of Salomon Brothers, Inc. figures that the rich HMO's have enough cash to buy up every advertising minute on Superbowl telecasts to run their commercials for the next 136 years. "It is way, way beyond what HMO's need" to meet insurance industry requirements, she added. In spite of the huge reserves and not knowing what to do with it, one financially strong HMO in New York is wasting clients and taxpayers money on legal costs going to court to plead for a rate increase which was initially denied.

Rate increases are not justified in many instances. A large company with 76,000 employees, half of which are enrolled in HMO's or other managed care programs, was able to negotiate a 15 percent rate reduction from the HMO for fiscal 1995. Other companies are banding together to demand relief of 5–10 percent or more from other HMO's.

Instead of giving all those premium dollars to HMO's who don't even know where to put the money, we must move quickly to establish medical savings plan options that allow employees to put these excess dollars into their own individual medical savings plan. It should be abundantly clear that people who have worked 15–20 years will have sufficient money in their medical savings account and will not need government assistance or company-sponsored retiree medical insurance to protect them at a later date. This would be the single most effective tool to save Medicare from certain bankruptcy, especially when "baby boomers" soon become Medicare beneficiaries.

Insurance companies must lead the way to bring about true health care reform that brings down the cost for everybody with a reasonable profit for both the insurance industry and providers. However, if they continue to extract maximum concessions from providers, pocket the big profits and buy up other companies, the free market will again make further cost reduction decisions for them on very unfavorable terms. They will certainly force industry to make their own arrangements and physicians may wake up and begin to assert themselves instead of taking whatever the payers dish out. Many large and medium size corporations are doing just that—making direct deals with providers, lab and pharmaceutical companies and cutting out the middle man.

CHAPTER 7

The Agenda For Health Care Reform: Putting Solutions Into Action

Senators Harris Wofford of Pennsylvania and J. Robert Kerrey of Nebraska deserve special recognition for championing health care issues long before it became glamorous.

President and Mrs. Clinton have succeeded in bringing the health care issue to the country's top agenda and should be commended for having the courage to do what others have shied away from. The President should also be commended for stating categorically that he is flexible and willing to seriously consider any proposal that offers universal coverage and reduces costs. On close analysis, the recommendations of the President's advisors probably would legislate universal coverage, but eventually would have great difficulty controlling costs and consequently be unable to deliver all the promised benefits. His plan and many others do not deal adequately with the fundamental causes of the explosive rise in medical costs and lack of needed access.

On the issue of reducing costs, these facts should be kept in mind:

1. One percent of the population consumes nearly 30 percent of our health care dollars.
2. Five percent consume 58 percent of our resources.
3. Ten percent consume fully 75 percent of health care funds.
4. The healthiest 50 percent of Americans are responsible for only three percent of health care spending or consumption.

The large segment of the American population who are fortunate enough to be in good health, who also choose a healthy lifestyle and avoid self-destructive behavior should have some money left over from their "share of the pie" to save for their own possible future medical needs. They do not deserve to be excessively taxed to pay for the care of 10 percent of the population, especially since at least 25 percent of the health care dollars are misallocated and can be made readily available to care for the uninsured. There is no implication here that the only reason for ill health is lifestyle. One can do all the right things and yet be struck by devastating illness.

On the issue of providing universal coverage, the following facts define the problem:

1. Approximately 15 percent of Americans are uninsured or underinsured.

2. More than half of uninsured people are in between jobs and the temporary lack of insurance might last anywhere from four to twelve months.

3. It has been demonstrated by other health care systems in which universal coverage is offered that approximately five percent of the population will not use the benefits even though they are available to them.

4. Therefore, the number of people chronically uninsured who would utilize available health care is actually three to four percent with approximately another seven percent who are temporarily uninsured.

The solutions for these two groups (the temporarily and chronically uninsured) *must* be different because of the fundamental differences in the reasons for the lack of coverage.The proposals we will outline here will make health care available to those who need it, reduce excessive and inappropriate spending and put some money in the pockets of most American families who help to control their own medical costs. All of this can be accomplished while maintaining the excellent features of our current health care system which has become the envy of the rest of the world. We can achieve this without employer mandates or an increase in either disguised or frank taxes.

First of all, we must appreciate the difficulty the lawmakers face in crafting a plan that can accomplish cost reduction, provide coverage for everyone and, at the same time, win votes at home. There are more than a dozen proposals with new ones cropping up nearly every week. It is becoming evident from the diverse array of plans being tossed about Washington that there is no cohesive plan or bipartisan approach forthcoming.

Many of our leaders are afraid to commit to any concrete idea for fear it might draw politically damaging "heat" from some particular group. These various lobbying groups who are concerned about protecting their own interests in the reform process have already spent $100 million. We are offering lawmakers a way out by suggesting a set of plans that have worked and can easily be adapted to achieve the national goals we all desire.

Over the past five years, industry has demanded and is already finding solutions to the health care crisis. We previously discussed the progress Rochester, New York and Cleveland, Ohio have made in reducing hospital costs. Cleveland's ranking as the fourth most expensive city in the nation was dropped to 19th, in terms of hospital costs, from 1985 to 1991. Nationwide, the hospital inflation rate rose by 8.3 percent in 1991, while Cleveland's rate of increase was only 4.4 percent. The rapid improvement was due in part to a state law passed in 1987 which allowed commercial insurance companies to negotiate with hospitals for better prices.

What needs to be done is to follow these kinds of examples and implement the salient features that make them successful instead of embarking on wholesale government intervention and disruption of the system. Senator John Chafee's remarks vocalized the concerns of many in a March 17, 1994 article in *Christian Science Monitor.* "...Whenever government gets involved in economic or social problems the costs go way beyond what you originally anticipated and therefore you have to be terribly cautious." As one of the authors of the Medicare program once remarked, health care is 20 percent legislation and 80 percent implementation.

As we have pointed out in chapter 5, most of the health care programs in other industrial countries are in serious trouble because of high costs and lack of money to finance what has been promised to the population. We must pay attention to *what is already working* and incorporate these ideas into the current health care reform. What we propose in this book will systematically control costs without turning the system upside down or inflicting any more economic hardship on individuals or corporations.

PRIORITY I. REDUCING EXCESSIVE COSTS

Before tackling the problems of availability of coverage and access to health care, we will reiterate some of the important elements in reducing health care costs. There are three key players in the health care cost crisis whose participation in reform must be solicited simultaneously. The successful control of these three elements will completely and virtually eliminate the health care crisis in terms of cost. If we seriously pay attention to these areas, *not a single dime of taxes needs to be raised.*

Malpractice reform, modifying doctors' practice patterns and changing the behavior of the consumer are all equally important. These three factors must be controlled simultaneously as the control of one hinges upon the control of the other. As the ultimate purchasers of health care services, individuals bear the responsibility of altering their behavior patterns from one of excessive utilization to using health care prudently and economically. Patients must be given incentives to help control their own costs. Without the cooperation of consumers, no effort to control costs will be totally successful.

The major responsibility for reducing unnecessary care and over utilization lies with doctors, regardless of what factors induce them to perform unnecessary services that drive up the costs.

Malpractice reform is pivotal to any efforts to reduce excessive procedures. We cannot ignore the domino effect of our current legal system on health care spending.

Participation of Lawyers in Health Care Reform

Malpractice reform must be a true reform and not a window dressing. We have described the severity of the current situation and discussed the solutions in considerable detail in Chapter Four. The backbone of reform should include a California-type solution, but must go much further and also include a cap on attorney's fees as suggested by several plans in Congress. An appropriate cap will leave a substantial amount of the award to the injured and, at the same time, adequately reward the attorney. Senator Cooper's plan limits lawyers' fees to 25 percent of the first $150,000 of the award and 10 percent of the remainder. This concept should be carried further so that all of the award in excess of $1 million goes to the injured party. In this way, the injured receive ample compensation, the attorney is well paid and the incentive to seek excessively large awards has been removed.

An effort should also be made to diminish the expenses to the lawyer by providing, for example, a panel of competent, fair expert witnesses at a reasonable cost. Expert witnesses must be truly experts in their field. Unqualified, "hired guns" should be outlawed.

There should be a stricter penalty for those who are continuously filing frivolous lawsuits with the hope of making easy money through coercive settlements. Some insurance companies' preference to settle, to avoid costly legal battles, has left them open to cases without merit.

We need stricter controls on incompetent physicians, as well. These physicians should be asked to seek proper help or if they are unwilling or continuously fail to make the grade, they should be effectively restrained to protect patients. Special exemptions or low cost malpractice premiums should be made available to volunteering nurses and doctors. Such a provision would enable those who have retired and solely want to volunteer their time and talents to do so.

A cost-effective means of arbitration or alternative conflict resolution for medical-legal conflicts must be firmly established. Arbitration results should be binding with a few clearly defined exceptions. If the client and the lawyer reject the arbitration decision and they lose, they should pay the court costs and legal fees of the winner. Very importantly, awards for pain and suffering should be more standardized. Other sources of compensation, such as expenses paid by insurance should be considered in determining the amount of the award.

Participation of Doctors in Health Care Reform

Alter Patient Care Patterns: Eliminate Excesses. Since doctors are responsible for ordering the vast majority of all procedures, they must also accept the responsibility of making the most beneficial choices in treating their patients to curb excessive use of tests and technology. The three major reasons for over-utilization which we have explored in great detail are: fear of lawsuits, the ingrained behavior patterns resulting from early training of doctors to do all possible tests and procedures that are needed to distinguish a particular diagnosis, and patient demand to receive specific tests and x-rays.

Most people believe that the reason why doctors order so many tests is because they receive some financial gain from those tests. While this may be true to some extent, the majority of tests ordered are performed by the hospital or laboratory without the doctor receiving any financial benefit whatsoever. For example, when a doctor admits a patient to the hospital or performs most outpatient evaluations, all the tests which are ordered do not benefit the doctor. The radiologist, who interprets these x-rays for a fee, is not happy when too many unnecessary tests are ordered. Although the radiologists are the ones who benefit from excessive x-ray testing, they are the most vocal critics of doctors who order too many tests.

We must be very careful, however, not to confuse admonition for over-utilization with the concept of rationing. Rationing always has a negative image in relation to health care because of the suggestion of limiting the care we provide. Sometimes, however, limiting care is far better than continuing care that is useless and sometimes outright damaging to the patient.

Peer Review: On-Site, Binding Procedural Decision-Making. The benefits of an on-site, impartial peer review board, as discussed in Chapter 3, would be invaluable in helping to ensure better patient care decisions. This board of specially trained and highly skilled physicians and nurses would be paid from monies contributed by hospitals and all insurance companies, including Medicare, to act in the best interest of all parties. The cost would be only a tiny fraction of the current arrangement of funding concurrent and post-care review in every department at every hospital, as well as every insurance organization doing their own review. This process would save the insurance industry huge sums of money and at the same time reduce the administrative hassle and nightmarish interference and burden on doctors. For example, a 54-year-old orthopedic doctor from Peoria, Illinois, had to employ one full time nurse to deal with the insurance companies because of the constant hassles. Yet he still spends about an hour to an hour and a half each day talking to out of town insurance nurse reviewers to justify why a particular patient is still in the hospital. He has to give details of the urine output, blood pressure, antibiotic dose, IV fluid rate and treatment plans to get one or two extra days approved for the patient to stay in the hospital and this process begins all over again in about 24 to 48 hours.

The role of an in-house review board could also be extended to the outpatient setting. Currently, there is no effective method of policing doctors locally when they perform their services outside the hospital. This peer review board could eventually have jurisdiction or oversight responsibility for problems related to excessive overutilization outside the hospital. Their scope would be truly limited to real or potential problems and not cause undue interference in the daily activities of doctors as the insurance companies are currently doing. These peer review panels must have sufficient legal protection and clout to do their work effectively. This process would also lead to collection of sufficient data to identify and significantly curtail unnecessary and overutilized procedures.

Participation of Individuals in Health Care Reform

As we have previously discussed, there is a tremendous imbalance in health care consumption, which is fairly unique to this country, in that one percent of the sickest patients consume nearly 30 percent of the health care dollars. Some of these people are simply unfortunate to develop serious illness beyond their control. Extremely sophisticated high tech treatment is also responsible for some of the imbalance. A large portion of this disparity, however, is due to the fact that a poor standard of living and certain lifestyles have a negative impact on the health of individuals.

Every attempt should be made to encourage and persuade people to give up costly behavior patterns such as smoking, alcohol and drug abuse, and poor exercise and eating habits. Smoking is the number one preventable cause of illness and premature death in this country. The danger is not only to those who choose to smoke, but also to those who live and work with the smoker. In the 90's, smoking-related deaths will account for about one-fourth of all deaths in developed countries for people age 35 to 70.

Joe Califano, former Secretary of Health, Education and Welfare under President Carter, has called an attack on smoking and other substance abuse crucial to health care reform. He stated that a minimum of $140 billion of our $1 trillion health care bill can be attributed to substance abuse. This estimate does not even include secondary costs, such as care for victims of accidents caused by drunk drivers. (*Christian Science Monitor*, 3/23/94)

Most experts believe that if we can help kids get through their teenage years without smoking, it would significantly reduce the number of people who smoke since 90 percent of smokers start the habit as teens.

Government's Role in Fostering Health Care Reform

The role of government should be quite limited in some areas of health care reform. The government should not take control of the health care system, largely because of the poor track record demonstrated with Medicare and Medicaid. Coverage under Medicare and Medicaid continues to diminish every year in futile attempts to keep costs down. The sheer magnitude of bureaucracy that would be required to administer a government-run program for the entire country would render the system unwieldy and ineffective from the outset.

There are other significant areas, however, where the government is needed to play a major part in bringing health care costs down—namely, reducing unemployment and enacting laws fostering conditions that enable people to individually own their insurance rather than having insurance tied to their job. Importantly, the insurance industry should not be allowed to restrict coverage because of pre-existing conditions, which is one thing everybody seems to agree on.

Anti-Poverty Campaign: Educate, Train, Provide Opportunity. Job loss is one of the single most important factors contributing to ill health and lack of insurance in this country. Government must do everything it can to create more jobs and help people find jobs that they are qualified to perform. This would also help reduce welfare dependency. Providing a climate that is conducive to high employment and reduces dependence on welfare would help foster the control of health care costs. The concept of reforming the unemployment system to a re-employment system with training, counseling, centralized access to data, and whatever other aid is needed to help the unemployed land a job, is a step in the right direction.

The Clinton administration should be congratulated for exemplary performance in job creation, i.e., two million jobs each year so far. However, the high rate of new job creation is being negated by huge job loss through company downsizing. This will continue and might accelerate if companies continue to spend 50 percent or more of after-tax profit on health care. Savings in health care outlay for businesses will lead to economic expansion and more jobs. This is why it is essential that any sensible health care reform package should not increase taxes on companies or individuals.

Making health care coverage available is only part of the equation for solving the problems of the uninsured. Widespread poverty and violence are major stumbling blocks to providing access to care and reducing costs. A major part of the government's role is to seriously attack the escalation of poverty and violence.

The recently promoted idea of "three strikes, you're out" is a poor solution to the violence problem because it does not address the main causes of violence and poverty but only fights the symptoms. It takes huge sums of money from the taxpayers to lock up a large segment of people who could be trained and educated to become productive and useful citizens if the funds and opportunities were available. The amateur criminals will be locked up while career or hard core criminals, rapists, serial killers and violent drug pushers continue to roam the streets. It is important to lock up dangerous criminals who are a menace to themselves and to society, but a wholesale construction of more jails and spending billions to lock up people is a gross misuse of scarce resources, especially when it depletes the funds available for education, health care, and productive employment. Advocating "three strikes, you're out" makes the lawmakers feel that they are tough on crime but, in fact, some segments of the current anti-crime laws will surely be tougher on the pocketbooks of the taxpayers than on hard core criminals.

PRIORITY II. COVERING THE UNINSURED AND UNDERINSURED

We have addressed at various stages in this book how the cost of providing health care for all can be reduced. Substantial reduction in the cost could be used to cover the less than seven percent of people who are chronically uninsured. The solution to providing coverage for everyone, therefore, is to reduce and control excessive costs, and thereby make the premium affordable for the uninsured.

Health Care Coverage for the Temporarily Uninsured

Let's deal first of all with the people who are temporarily uninsured or underinsured while in between jobs—approximately seven percent of Americans. Dr. George Fisher, M.D., an internist in Philadelphia who writes as a columnist for USA Today, states that of the nearly 40 million uninsured people, 30 million are in between jobs for an average time period of four months.

The "New COBRA." In order to take care of unemployed people who are in transit, I am proposing that modifications be made to the COBRA plan. Providing temporary coverage in this manner would not only be simple to implement, it would eliminate the need to tax small businesses or establish an employer mandate for health insurance. Larger businesses would get substantial benefit from other savings to compensate for providing these benefits. The cost of extending the employee's coverage for a few months with a modified COBRA plan at a reduced rate is small compared to the large annual health care premium increases now faced by businesses and the threat of new taxes on these premiums.

The plan would work like this: presently, when an employee loses their job they are allowed to participate in the former employer's plan at their own cost for about 18 months. Since the majority of people who lose their jobs are re-employed within a year or less, it would be reasonable to change the COBRA plan so that the former employer continues to cover the ex-employee with either a modified or comprehensive health care plan for a period of about 12 months. To qualify for the program, a reasonable minimum length of employment could be specified by the employer. A modified plan, similar to the one we described in Hollywood, Florida, would provide coverage at a cost of about one-third the average employer's current cost and help the insurance industry as well as the providers of health care. The cost of extending this coverage, about $150 to $250 per month for a family plan, could be borne by the employee alone or could be shared by the employer and the former employee. This arrangement would not be very costly for the employer and would guarantee coverage to protect the patient from catastrophic illness that would wipe out their life savings. The major reason why it has been difficult for the temporarily uninsured to have any decent coverage is government regulations. State regulations of the 1980's have made affordable premiums completely out of reach for individuals and small groups. The 1980's was the first decade which showed an increase in the uninsured population. This is directly related to the State legislators mandating the number and type of benefits which consumers are required to buy. Whether they need it, want it, or can afford it, they are compelled to have it. A taxi driver in New York can afford a "no-frills" insurance plan which would be more than adequate for him. However, he cannot afford a $450–$600 premium per month for a policy with all the mandated coverage. There were 40 million individual health policies in 1980. There are now 30 million because excessive regulations make the premiums unaffordable.

In the *Wall Street Journal,* February 28, 1994, Elizabeth McCaughey, a Health Policy Analyst at Manhattan Institute, proposed an excellent way to offer health care insurance to all families, no matter how little they can afford, in a manner that will not add a single dollar to the Federal budget. She says none of the health care proposals in Congress offers the kind of solution she has in mind and suggested that providing affordable, no-frills insurance for those who need it should be the first priority. Ms. McCaughey illustrates the detrimental effect of the 1980's legislation by pointing out some examples of costly mandated benefits such as alcohol abuse treatment required by 30 states, drug rehabilitation required by 20 states, coverage for chiropractic services required by 45 states, and even acupuncture coverage required by three states.

Ms. McCaughey stressed that keeping health care affordable is key to health care reform. Practically all uninsured adults are either between jobs or working at low wages and 75 percent are covered again within a year, usually through an employer. She states that what they need most during that transition period is low-cost protection not a "gold-plated policy" loaded with extras they cannot afford. Furthermore, she believes that even for those who can afford it, the gold-plated insurance is not necessarily better because it only encourages excessive usage.

She points out that the premium for a young person should be fairly affordable. Half of all the uninsured adults are under 30 years old. Ms. McCaughey suggests that a 25-year-old person needs coverage for less than $600 a year while a 55-year-old person on the average will need a $2400 annual premium in order to provide sufficient coverage. If health insurance premiums are too high, a 30-year-old person will simply not buy it.

She also believes that community pricing will result in a serious problem for young adults, citing a vivid example. In April 1993, New York mandated community pricing and saw an 80 percent jump in premium for people under 30 years old. The premium has also increased considerably for other segments such as small businesses who have seen their premiums increase by about 110 percent. The community pricing philosophy will clearly cause a big increase in premiums in inner cities and adjacent communities. These areas consume a disproportionate amount of the health care dollars. Community pricing could potentially cause hardships for a significant segment of the population. The five percent of the population who consume about 50 percent of health care dollars, probably congregate in these areas. A more cost-effective method would be to let people choose what coverage they need and what they can afford thus reducing the number of uninsured. Community rating does work, however, if it is carefully designed and implemented as in Rochester, New York, for example.

Health Care Coverage for the Chronically Uninsured

As things stand now, if we subtract the number of people who are uninsured because of transient layoff from the total uninsured population, we are left with about four to seven percent of Americans who are chronically uninsured. It is a fact that in all the other industrialized countries, even where universal coverage is provided, there are about five percent of the people who do not take advantage of the available health coverage unless they are in severe pain or near death. Therefore, in reality, we are only talking about paying for care for three to four percent of the population. This relatively small number of chronically uninsured should be incorporated into a re-organized Medicaid system.

The "New Medicaid": A Privatized System. Medicaid, as we now know it, should be totally dismantled and privatized along the same line as the Hollywood, Florida model or spread over other private insurance companies. To implement a privatized Medicaid system, patients should be assigned to a primary care physician and encouraged to follow up with their physician regularly. This would stop the current trend of small manageable illnesses becoming very advanced and requiring extensive care. This trend results in frequent emergency room visits and hospitalization. Insurance companies would be contracted to provide coverage at close to their cost and government funds would cover the cost of coverage for those who cannot afford to pay. Payment for coverage by others would be based on income level. By privatizing the Medicaid program the patient would be better accepted and more willing to seek adequate health care at an earlier stage when it would do the most good.

There are a lot of voluntary religious and not-for-profit health care organizations and hospitals that should be strengthened to help provide additional needed services. Community clinics need to be developed and expanded to serve the needs of patients more effectively. These clinics can be staffed by a combination of paid and volunteer nurses, nurse practitioners, social workers and doctors.

Community Clinics: Education, Access, Lower Cost Services. We can offer health care coverage to all but if we do not provide a means of getting the help when it is needed and educating people on the importance of getting proper care, then health care reform will fall short of one of its major tasks. There are a large number of practicing and retiring health care workers who would be willing to volunteer time to provide free service to patients.

A movie director from Hollywood, California states that his father, who is a 64-year-old surgeon, wants to retire but would like to continue to contribute his services in some way. However, he is unable to do so because he must carry malpractice insurance at a cost of $25,000 to $30,000 a year in order to be able to take care of socio-economically disadvantaged patients. There are thousands of doctors and nurses who have retired and no doubt would be willing to spend four to ten hours a week volunteering if we produce a facility and a climate conducive to community service.

Instead of relying exclusively on emergency room services, community clinics and hospital outpatient clinics provide needed care at a much more reasonable cost. The improper use of emergency rooms should be discouraged. Most people have some form of access to health care. However, they go to the wrong place for their care. Patients who make it a habit to come to the emergency room for routine care should be referred to family physicians or community clinics. As we discussed in chapter 5, the use of key health care professionals in a clinic in Canada enabled them to innovatively care for patients' needs and significantly reduce the number of re-visits to doctors offices. In addition, they were able to substantially reduce the amount of tranquilizers patients were consuming. Many of the illnesses patients suffer are a result of unemployment, stress and family problems that a five minute doctor's office visit with a prescription for Valium would certainly not alleviate. These types of problems are better dealt with in a community clinic with social service counselors, nurse practitioners and a supervising doctor as the need arises. In an interview by C. Burns Roehrig, M.D. reported in February, 1992, *Internist,* Louis W. Sullivan related that one of his major accomplishments was the revitalization of the National Health Service Corporation. He had resurrected it from $8 million in annual scholarship funds to a program of nearly $60 million. He added he hoped to increase it to nearly 4500 physicians by the year 2000. These doctors can man the inner city and rural clinics.

This type of approach would significantly reduce medical costs and the dependency on alcohol and drugs as a substitute for solving problems. Doctors and other health care providers would be willing to provide services at a reduced price, as shown in the example of the Hollywood, Florida system.

Volunteerism by health care providers can also be vital in improving compliance with important health care services such as vaccination. Poor vaccination rates nationwide have not improved even when vaccinations were provided free of charge. This is primarily due to lack of knowledge by the parents as to the importance of vaccination, as well as a need for improvement in access to the place of service. Nurse volunteers and social service workers could be instrumental in increasing the rate of vaccination and use vacant community health clinics, especially in the evenings, to improve the health of the children and the community at large. Throwing more money on government purchased vaccines will not improve the situation.

Medisave: The Life Saver

Of all the health care proposals, one idea that should have more prominence, but has not had the necessary publicity, is Medisave. This concept, which has already been tried, would put the consumer squarely in control of current cost and utilization, as well as the future security of their health care. The more closely we examine and explore the possibilities and advantages of the consumer being in charge of their own expenditure, the more exciting and appealing the idea becomes. It is truly a remarkable idea. The advantages are almost infinite and the disadvantages are almost nonexistent. Though still a low profile idea, more than a dozen plans now in Congress

The Medisave Advantage

$ Available For Premium	Premium Paid	Plan Deductible	Deductible Not Spent	Employer Year End Savings	Employee Year End Savings	Employee's 10 Yr Savings Account	Employee' 20 Yr Savings Account
$4500 Traditional Plan	$4500	$250	-0-	-0-	[-$250]	[-$4200]	[-$12,600]
$4500 Medisave Plan	$1500	$3000	$2000	$500	$1500	$23,500	$74,000
$6000 Traditional Plan	$6000	$250	-0-	-0-	[-$250]	[-$4200]	[-$12,600]
$6000 Medisave Plan	$1500	$3000	$2000	$1500	$2000	$31,300	$99,000

Above is an illustration of the Medisave Advantage for two employees enrolled in traditional health care plans with annual premiums of $4500 and $6000. The employee savings accounts reflect conservative estimates of a consistent annual year end benefit and an interest rate of 8%. The employer year end benefit reflects the cost of premium spent or the net savings resulting from reduced premium cost and/or a portion of the unspent deductible funds provided for the employee.

have some version of the Medisave concept with a combined total of about 200 co-sponsors. This has caused Michael Turner, an expert on health care issues, to state that Medisave is the most popular concept in Congress.

Health care premiums are really a portion of the salary of the employee. Unfortunately, since this money does not currently go directly to the employee, they have the mistaken notion that the premium is somebody else's money and therefore it should be used to the maximum without regard to cost. This type of behavior would change effectively with Medisave which makes it clear to the employee that the premium actually belongs to them.

The average health care premium is approximately $4500 with some as high as $6000 for companies with very extensive health benefit packages, like DuPont and Chrysler. By paying low premiums, for example $1500 with a high deductible of $3000, the patient has $3000 to $4500 available to pay for deductible expenses. If the patient spends only $1500 of this, he has $1500 to $3000 left to save or partially spend or to split the remainder between the employer and the employee. If an employee saves between $1500 to $2000 each year for the next 10 years, at eight percent interest he will have about $23,500 to $31,300. In 20 years, he will have $74,000 to $99,000. I realize Medisave is not a panacea for the health care crisis. If poorly implemented, Medisave could turn out to be a bonanza only for the wealthy, the healthy and a few insurance companies that only insure the healthy and hence, penalize companies that insure the sicker population. However, a properly designed Medisave coupled with prudent legal, insurance and practice pattern reforms will save well over $150 –$200 billion annually. It is absolutely certain that we can eliminate 20% of the services we provide to our patients and still improve the quality of care. Medisave is the best consumer incentive to eliminate unnecessary services and achieve overall cost reduction.

This is the only concept I have seen in the health care debate that would guarantee about 60 percent of Americans health care security. The sum of money they have accumulated could be transferred and used for coverage should they temporarily lose their job. This idea is particularly well-suited for America, where 50 percent of the population consumes only three percent of the health care dollars which means that a substantial number of people would be saving a considerable amount of money for current and future health care expenditures.

A government can give every person a plastic card but cannot guarantee benefits without taxation in some form. Yet this plastic card is no guarantee because as the government resources get leaner, the benefits would either get smaller or taxes would have to be raised, as we see in Canada, the United Kingdom and Germany, to maintain the same benefits.

If "baby boomers" begin to save money through a Medisave plan now, we can even save Medicare from expected bankruptcy. The widespread application of this Medisave concept will have immediate impact on reduction of the medical outlay and proponents estimate that it would reduce the cost of medical care by at least 25 percent. This concept is not intended to merely provide catastrophic coverage. Insurance companies can still make a handsome profit if Medisave is combined with the other two major cost reduction ideas presented in this book, namely, malpractice reform and controlling doctors' behavior. Furthermore, the consumer is the best instrument in detecting health care fraud, which is currently estimated to cost the system $100 billion.

The threat of health care reform has already produced some beneficial results, such as markedly reduced health care inflation, recently estimated at 8 percent. This has primarily been accomplished by large companies using their clout to squeeze providers to control costs and refusing to pay for uncompensated health care costs for the uninsured and those under-insured in government programs. Allowing these statistics to lull us into inaction on health care reform will ultimately make it more difficult for the uninsured to obtain care since providers can no longer shoulder the cost of uncompensated care. Patients will forestall treatment of medical problems until they are at a more critical stage resulting in higher costs, especially for federal and state governments. State and federal deficits will worsen. Health care costs for small businesses will rise causing more people to lose their jobs or work without health care coverage. As more middle-class Americans lose their jobs or insurance coverage, the clamor for employer mandates could become politically more powerful. Broad-based taxes will become unavoidable as government expenditures for health care increase.

The greatest problem now is complacency which may lead some to want to leave the system relatively unchanged. This would be a serious mistake with devastating consequences. Implementing a sensible and successful agenda for health care reform requires something from all of us. No one is blameless in the health care crisis and no one is exempt from responsibility in its solution.

A carefully orchestrated reform process incorporating the concepts we have discussed can foster elimination of wasteful spending through malpractice reform and changes in the behavior patterns of physicians and patients, as well as promote efficient and effective use of funds to make health care services available for all. If we can combine the beneficial effects of Medisave along with a strong malpractice reform and genuine cooperation from hospitals and doctors to do their part, there certainly would be more than enough money left to further reduce premiums and provide care for every American. The consequences of a lack of any action or the wrong actions are deep and far-reaching for our society, as a whole, and for our own personal well-being and the future standard of living for our children.

BIBLIOGRAPHY

INTRODUCTION

Samuelson, RJ. Health Care: How we got into this mess. *Newsweek* 1993 Oct 4;122(14):29-35.

Sullivan, LW. Louis W. Sullivan, MD: At the Helm in a Time of Reform. *The Internist.* 1992 Feb: 20-22.

Allen GH. A wake up call from C. Everett Koop, M.D. *Health Care News* 1993 May:5.

Merline J. Not everyone likes Clinton health reforms, businesses fear soaring costs, more government controls. *Investor's Business Daily* 1993 Sep 24.

CHAPTER 1

deLorimier AA (President American Pediatric Surgical Association). Health care costs in a declining America. *Journal of Pediatric Surgery.* 1993 Mar;28(3):281-91.

Barondess, JA, Ginzberg E, Blendon RJ, Inglehart J, Relman, AS, Aiken LH, participants. Medical economics in the 90's. Symposium at Cornell University Medical College 1992 May 16; New York City. *Cornell University Alumni Quarterly* 1993;53(1):2-12.

Samuelson RJ. Health Care: How we got into this mess. *Newsweek* 1993 Oct 4;122(14):29-35.

Merline J. How will health care reform work? *Investor's Business Daily* 1993 Dec 14;10(173):1-2.

Warden C. Letting employees rein in costs. *Investor's Business Daily* 1993 May 20;10(29):1-2.

Clements M. DuPont shifts burden onto employees. *USA Today* 1993 Mar 12:1B-2B.

Couch JB. The potential role of corporate America in ameliorating the medial liability problem. *Legal Medicine* 1990:243-60.

Reuters. Can retirees count on medical coverage anymore? *Investor's Business Daily.*

Cigna Insight, 2nd qtr 1993;2(2):2.

McGivney WT. Biotechnology: Will it break the health care bank? *Physician Executive* 1992 Sep-Oct;18(5):35-6.

Rising prescription drug prices. *Internist* 1992 Oct:45.

Pricing pain: Relief in sight on drug costs? *Journal of American Health Policy* 1992 Nov-Dec:28-31.

Terry K. How much preventive care can we afford? *Medical Economics* 1993 Aug 23.

Toner R. How much health care reform will the patient go along with? *New York Times* 1993 Mar.

Angell, M. How much will health care reform cost? *New England Journal of Medicine* 1993 Jun 17:1778-9.

CHAPTER 2

Samuelson RJ. Health Care: How we got into this mess. *Newsweek* 1993 Oct 4;122(14):29-35.

Barondess, JA, Ginzberg E, Blendon RJ, Inglehart J, Relman, AS, Aiken LH, participants. Medical economics in the 90's. Symposium at Cornell University Medical College 1992 May 16; New York City. *Cornell University Alumni Quarterly* 1993;53(1):2-12.

Increase in health benefit costs eased to 8% for firms in 1993. *Investor's Business Daily* 1994 Feb 15:3.

Sperry P. High-tech medicine's high cost. *Investor's Business Daily* 1993 May 25:1-2.

Deutschman DA. Rationing: A mindless paradox buttressed by our deepest fears. *Cleveland Physician.*

Merline J. Will reform keep you healthy? Investor's Business Daily 1993 May 13.

Hansagi H, et al. High consumers of health care in emergency units: How to improve their quality of care. *Quality Assurance in Health Care* 1991;3(1):51-62.

Norbeck TB. Rising health care costs: Disease or symptom? *Connecticut Medicine.* v57:235-7.

Sullivan, LW. Louis W. Sullivan, MD: At the Helm in a Time of Reform. *The Internist* 1992 Feb: 20-22.

Bartecchi, CE, et al. The Human Costs of Tobacco Use (First of Two Parts). *The New England Journal of Medicine.* 1994 Mar 31: 907-912.

MacKenzie TD, et al. The Human Costs of Tobacco Use (Second of Two Parts). *The New England Journal of Medicine.* 1994 Apr 7: 975-980.

Sullivan, LW. Family Physicians and a Smoke-Free Society. *American Family Physician.* 1990 Nov:1453-1456.

Applebome P. CDC's new chief worries as much about bullets as about bacteria. *New York Times* 1993 Sep 26.

Oliver C. Why do kids become criminals? *Investor's Business Daily* 1993 Dec 20.

Study: 21% rise in HIV treatment costs by 1994. *Hospitals* 1992 Jan 20.

Black RF, Collins S, Boroughs DL. The hidden cost of AIDS. *U.S. News & World Report* 1992 Jul 27:48-59.

Hellinger F. Blue Cross Blue Shield Association. *Inquiry* 1991.

Terry K. How much preventive care can we afford? *Medical Economics* 1993 Aug 23:124-35.

Woolhandler S, et al. Administrative costs in U.S. hospitals. *New England Journal of Medicine* 1993 Aug 5;329(6):400-3.

Stevens C. Will administrative savings really pay for health care reform? *Medical Economics* 1993 Oct 25:147-54.

Stroud M. High-tech fix for health care? *Investor's Business Daily.*

Woolhandler S, Himmelstein D. Deteriorating administrative efficiency of the U.S. health care system. *New England Journal of Medicine* 1991 May 2:1253-8.

Hanlon CR. The second opinion. *CA—A Cancer Journal for Clinicians* 1978 Nov-Dec;28(6):363-6.

Ashby JL, Lisk CK. Why do hospital costs continue to increase? *Health Affairs* 1992 Summer:134-47.

Warden C. Should government cover everyone? *Investor's Business Daily* 1994 Jan 10:1-2.

Merline J. Who pays for our health care? *Investor's Business Daily* 1993 Sep 7:1-2.

Ashby JL. The burden of uncompensated care grows. *Healthcare Financial Management* 1992 Apr:66-8.

Koop CE. Commencement Address to Cornell College Class of 1992.

CHAPTER 3

How doctors would cure the health care crisis. *Medical Economics* 1992 Sep 21:41-108.

Winawer SJ, et al. Randomized comparison of surveillance intervals after colonoscopic removal of newly diagnosed adenomatous polyps. *New England Journal of Medicine* 1993 Apr 1;328(13):901-6.

Jancin B. In-hospital CPR: High cost, low yield. *Internal Medicine News & Cardiology News* 1993 Jun 1.

Levy D. Call to give up on some cardiac cases. *USA Today* 1993 Sep 22.

Bernstein SJ, et al. The appropriateness of hysterectomy. *Journal of the American Medical Association* 1993 May 12;269(18):2398-2402.

Special report: The economics of Cancer. *Oncology Times* 1981 Nov.

Kapoor WN, et al. Syncope of unknown origin. *Journal of the American Medical Association* 1992 May 21;247(19):2687-91.

Brook RH, et al. Appropriateness of acute medical care for the elderly: An analysis of the literature. *Health Policy* 1990 Feb;14:225-42.

Alper PR. Why is it so hard to quit care that is futile? *Internal Medicine World Report* 1993 Mar 15.

Study questions life-prolonging acts in severe cancer cases. *New York Times* 1993 Feb 10:A12.

Holoweiko M. Hospital peer review: not just for bad apples anymore. *Medical Economics* 1991 Aug 19:150-64.

UR: From cost cutting to managing care. *Business & Health* 1993 Sep:41-4.

White O. This could end the rural doctor shortage. *Medical Economics* 1993 Dec 13:42-9.

Rosenthal E. Insurers second-guess doctors, provoking debate over savings. *New York Times* 1993 Jan 24:1.

Stevens C. Are clouds closing in on the Rochester miracle? *Medical Economics* 1993 Apr 25:106-23.

Burry J. Stop the waste. *Blue Cross & Blue Shield of Ohio* 1993 Summer;1(2):10-1.

Pollock EJ. Breast cancer diagnosis suits are increasing. *Wall Street Journal* 1993 Jul 22:B1-2.

Ingwerson M. Florida tests health care reform. *The Christian Science Monitor* 1993 May 6:3.

CHAPTER 4

Holoweiko M. What are your greatest malpractice risks? *Medical Economics* 1992 Aug 3:141-59.

Stein RS. Lawyers: The new racketeers? *Investor's Business Daily* 1994 Apr 4:1-2.

Stein RS. Has tort reform disappeared? *Investor's Business Daily* 1993 Dec 3:1-2.

Huber PW. How lawyers have invaded the delivery room. *Medical Economics* 1992 Dec 7:149-60.

Norland CC. Liability epidemic—health care costs: Break the linkage. *Missouri Medicine* 1992 Apr;89(4):226-30.

Brandt RI. The suit was frivolous, but I was trapped anyway. *Medical Economics* 1993 Sep 13:38-48.

Weaver K. The tort system's influence on the cost of health care. *The Internist* 1991 Oct:28-9.

Crane M. America's health crisis—the Dx—and the Rx. *Medical Economics* 1992 Sep 21:62-4.

Baumgartner A. The difference between physicians and attorneys. *Cleveland Physician.*

Kellar JR. How I survived six malpractice suits. *Medical Economics* 1992 Mar 16:165-74.

Crane M. How a hired gun's lies caught up with him. *Medical Economics* 1992 Aug 3:42-9.

Sharzer S. Defensive medicine is worthless—on two counts. *Medical Economics* 1993 Mar 22:41-8.

Lyons B. I blew my stack—and ended a malpractice ordeal. *Medical Economics* 1992 Dec 7:89-93.

Rice B. Where those expert witnesses come from. *Medical Economics* 1993 Jul 12:49-59.

Lerer RJ. It's not just plaintiff's experts who fudge the truth. *Medical Economics* 1994 May 23:27-34.

Crane M. Why hired guuns get away with lies. *Medical Economics* 1993 Dec 27:22-30.

McCann B. Malpractice premiums expected to go down. *Healthcare News* 1993 Sep:5.

Burg B. Isn't there something better than suing? *Medical Economics* 1992 Jul 6:164-95.

Goldfarb B. Arbitrating malpractice disputes. *Impact* 1994 Feb;2(2).

CHAPTER 5

Warden C. How U.S. health care stacks up. *Investor's Business Daily* 1993 Apr 29:1-2.

Sterngold J. Japan's health care: Cradle, grave and no frills. *New York Times* 1992 Dec 28:A1.

Barondess, JA, Ginzberg E, Blendon RJ, Inglehart J, Relman, AS, Aiken LH, participants. Medical economics in the 90's. Symposium at Cornell University Medical College 1992 May 16; New York City. *Cornell University Alumni Quarterly* 1993;53(1):2-12.

Farnsworth CH. Now patients are paying amid Canadian cutbacks. *New York Times* 1993 Mar 7:1.

Montgomery L. Can Canadian-style health care help us get Canadian-style malpractice? *NCMJ* 1992 Feb;53(2):100-4.

Azevedo D. Canada, the truth about queues. *Medical Economics* 1993 Feb 24:168-83.

Harper T. What can we learn from Europe. *Medical Economics* 1993 Sep 13:138-50.

Gammon M. Among Britain's ills, a health care crisis. *Internal Medicine World Report* 1993 Oct 15:4-5.

York, G. Fee-for-service: Cashing in on the Canadian medical care system. *Journal of Public Health Policy* 1992 Summer:140-5.

Salloum S, Franssen E. Laboratory investigations in general practice. *Canadian Family Physician* 1993 May;39:1055-61.

Morganthau T, Thomas R, Solomon J. The Clinton health papers. *Newsweek* 1993 Sep 20:30-37.

A summary of the Health Security Act of 1993. *Internal Medicine News & Cardiology News* 1993 Oct 15:19.

Appel A. Capitol Hill split over the health care bills. *The Christian Science Monitor* 1994 Mar 17:3.

Ingwerson M. Dueling health plans. *The Christian Science Monitor* 1994 Feb 16:7.

Warden C. Letting employees rein in costs. *Investor's Business Daily* 1990 May 2:1-2.

Merline J. Employees as health care reformers. *Investor's Business Daily* 1994, Mar 18:1-2.

CHAPTER 6

Anders G. HMO's pile up billions in cash, try to decide what to do with it. *Wall Street Journal* 1994 Dec 21:A1, A12.

Crane M. The malpractice dragon wasn't dead—just asleep. *Medical Economics* 1994 Oct 24:52-59.

Jancin B. Insurance companies spreading risks—but not profits—to doctors. *Internal Medicine News & Cardiology News* 1994 Dec 1:28.

Leavenworth, G. Four cost-cutting strategies. *Business & Health* 1994 Aug:26-33.

Murray D. Continuing survey: PPO's and HMO's. *Medical Economics* 1994 Nov 21:117-129.

Slomski A. How business is flattening health costs. *Medical Economics* 1994 Jul 11:87-100.

SoRell R. Future uncertain for MD Anderson. *Oncology Times* 1994 Dec:8-9.

Wood A.P. Managed care survey downplays role of physician disenrollment. *Internal Medicine News & Cardiology News* 1994 Dec 1:4.

Young R.C. Health care reform in the private sector. *Oncology Times* 1994 Dec;16 (12):2.

CHAPTER 7

Norbeck T. Rising health care costs: Disease or symptom? *Connecticut Medicine* 1993;57:235-7.

Bove VM. Health care costs tied to many issues. *Physician Executive* 1992 Sep-Oct;18(5):23-9.

Koop CE. Inject reality into children's health plan. *Plain Dealer* 1993 Feb:6C.

Warden C. When is a tax not a real tax? Budget scoring on mandates will drive debate. *Investor's Business Daily* 1994 Feb 1:1-2.

Warden C. Paying up for Clinton's reforms. *Investor's Business Daily* 1994 Jan 19:1-2.

Burry J. Squeezing cost out of the system. *Chief Executive* 1994 Jan-Feb.

Merline J. How will health care reform work? *Investor's Business Daily* 1993 Dec 14:1-2.

Trumbull M. Washington state: National lab on crime. *The Christian Science Monitor.*

Oliver C. Are more prisons the answer? *Investor's Business Daily* 1994 Jan 18:1-2.

Malkin J. Is "3 strikes, you're out" safe? *Investor's Business Daily* 1994 Mar 7:1-2.

Phillips L. Plenty of prisoners but not enough money. *USA Today* 1994 Mar 18:9A.

Blendon RJ, Greer Jr PJ, Angell M, Fisher GR. Is president's plan too bureaucratic? *USA Today* 1994 Mar 29:9A.

Hays K. Clinton package places small businesses in line of fire. *Investor's Business Daily* 1993 Jul 26:3.

McCann B. Malpractice premiums expected to go down. *Healthcare News* 1993 Sep:5.

Warden C. Other paths to health reform. *Investor's Business Daily* 1993 May 4:1-2.

Warden C. Passing the health care buck. *Investor's Business Daily* 1993 Apr 26:1-2.

Sullivan, LW. Louis W. Sullivan, MD: At the Helm in a Time of Reform. *The Internist* 1992 Feb: 20-22.

Trumbull M. Conservatives propose Medisave health care. *The Christian Science Monitor* 1994 Apr 5:2.

Fisher GR. Why not try these health reform ideas? *USA Today*.

Baquet C. The American health security plan. *National Medical Association News* 1993 Fall:2.

Rostenkowski stands by taxes for universal health coverage. *Investor's Business Daily* 1994 May 11.

Warden C. Letting employees rein in costs. *Investor's Business Daily* 1993 May 20:1-2.

Clements M. Health plan savings tip: Don't use it. *USA Today*.

Merline J. Employees as health reformers. *Investor's Business Daily* 1994 Mar 18:1-2.

Merline J. The cost of health reforms could reach $106 billion by 2000. *Investor's Business Daily* 1993 Dec 9.

Steele RJ. There's no quick fix for our health care system. *Medical Economics* 1992 Aug 3.

Stevens C. Are clouds closing in on the Rochester miracle? *Medical Economics* 1993 Apr 26:106-23.